A CONCISE ENCYCLOPEDIA
OF WOMEN'S SEXUAL
AND REPRODUCTIVE HEALTH

A CONCISE ENCYCLOPEDIA
OF WOMEN'S SEXUAL
AND REPRODUCTIVE HEALTH

Deborah Mitchell

A Lynn Sonberg Book

St. Martin's Paperbacks

Notice: This book is intended as a reference volume only, not as a medical manual. The information given here is designed to help you make informed decisions about your health. It is not intended as a substitute for any treatment that may have been prescribed by your doctor. If you suspect that you have a medical problem, we urge you to seek competent medical help.

Mention of specific companies, organizations, or authorities in the book does not imply endorsement by the author or publisher, nor does mention of specific companies, organizations, or authorities imply that they endorse this book, its author, or the publisher.

Internet addresses given in this book were accurate at the time it went to press.

A CONCISE ENCYCLOPEDIA OF WOMEN'S SEXUAL AND REPRODUCTIVE HEALTH

Copyright © 2009 by Lynn Sonberg Book Associates.

Cover photo © Burke / Triolo / Brand X Pictures / Jupiterimages.

For information address St. Martin's Press, 175 Fifth Avenue, New York, NY 10010.

ISBN: 978-1-250-06220-8

St. Martin's Paperbacks edition / March 2009

St. Martin's Paperbacks are published by St. Martin's Press, 175 Fifth Avenue, New York, NY 10010.

P1

TABLE OF CONTENTS

PART II: Tests, Surgeries, Procedures, and Devices

PART III: Getting What You Need: Quality Health Care

INTRODUCTION

You are holding in your hands a comprehensive, A-to-Z guide to women's reproductive and sexual health issues. It's been designed to help women of all ages be better informed both as health care consumers and as individuals who have questions about their reproductive and sexual health—from the onset of menstruation to postmenopause, pregnancy, sexually transmitted diseases, and how to choose a gynecologist and midwife.

My goal in writing this book is to bring together in one convenient, easy-to-read volume the latest, most authoritative information on women's reproductive and sexual health issues—information that until now was available only from many different sources. Chances are you picked up this book because you are much too busy to take the time to comb through all those sources: you need the information at your fingertips so that you can take responsibility not only for achieving optimal health but also for enjoying your life as a woman to the fullest.

One of the joys and challenges of being a woman is that your health care needs are always changing. Sometimes it may seem like you can barely keep up! Fortunately, there are many resources available to help you meet your needs and answer your questions. This book can address the questions you may have about a specific condition, symptom, or medical procedure, plus it brings together a wealth of resources that allow you to enhance your knowledge and help you make decisions about your health care concerns.

HOW TO USE THIS BOOK

To accomplish this goal we have presented information in a portable, encyclopedic format that's been divided into three parts, each with entries that are arranged A to Z and that are complete within themselves, but which also often provide cross-references to entries elsewhere in the book.

Part I includes entries covering reproductive and sexual diseases and conditions ranging from amenorrhea and infertility to premature ovarian failure and vaginal yeast infections. Each entry follows a fairly standard format, but there are a few variations depending on the information available. With that in mind, we include introductory information about the condition as well as risk factors and causes, symptoms, how a diagnosis is made, prevention and treatment options you can expect to hear about from your gynecologist and/or other involved health care professional, self-care and complementary approaches, and sources of additional information, including references to current research. Part I concludes with a Q&A segment.

Part II includes entries that cover medical tests, procedures, devices, and surgeries women may encounter in the realm of reproductive and sexual health. Topics range from abortion to cryosurgery, in vitro fertilization, and ultrasound. Once again, each entry follows a format and includes (as applicable) an explanation of the topic, how it is performed, how to prepare for it, benefits, risks and side effects, and sources of additional information. Again, a Q&A segment also follows the entries.

Part III brings together guidelines you can use to help you find the best possible health care for your reproductive and sexual health issues, whether you are looking for a gynecologist, a reproductive endocrinologist, or a midwife. This section also offers information that allows you to better understand and utilize the enormous wealth of health information available to all of us from print, the airwaves, cyberspace, and face-to-face sources.

PART I

Reproductive and Sexual Diseases and Conditions

AMENORRHEA

The absence of menstruation during puberty or later in a woman's life is called amenorrhea. This condition occurs in two forms, primary and secondary amenorrhea. The absence of menstruation and secondary sexual characteristics (pubic hair, breast development) in females by age fourteen or the absence of menstruation with normal development of secondary sexual characteristics in girls by age sixteen is primary amenorrhea. This affects less than 3 percent of adolescent girls. Females who were menstruating but then stop for three consecutive months or longer have secondary amenorrhea. Some experts qualify this definition by excluding the cessation of menstruation associated with pregnancy, lactation, use of birth control pills, or menopause; however, the first definition is the one more commonly used. Secondary amenorrhea is much more common than the primary form and typically is not serious.

Amenorrhea is a symptom of an underlying condition (see "Causes and Risk Factors") rather than a disease, and so additional symptoms may occur depending on what that condition is. Symptoms often associated with amenorrhea include headache, milky discharge from the nipples, hot flashes, sleep problems, severe anxiety, and excessive hair growth on the face and/or torso.

CAUSES AND RISK FACTORS

For some adolescent girls, the cause of primary amenorrhea is unknown. The most common reasons are heredity, poor nutrition, or an endocrine problem (e.g., hypothyroidism or a pituitary tumor). Other causes include a hormonal imbalance, eating disorders (e.g., anorexia nervosa, bulimia), extreme obesity, and excessive exercise. Young girls who take part in intensive physical training prior to puberty, which is common among gymnasts and ballet dancers, can delay the start of menstruation by up to five months for every year of training they have done.

Secondary amenorrhea may be caused by many of the same factors associated with the primary form, although the most common cause of secondary amenorrhea is pregnancy. Other causes include lactation, the use of certain medications (e.g., antidepressants, antipsychotics, chemotherapy drugs), chronic illness, uterine fibroids, premature menopause, use of birth control pills, menopause, and polycystic ovary syndrome.

DIAGNOSIS

To determine the cause of amenorrhea, your health care provider may run blood tests to determine the levels of hormones secreted by the ovaries (estrogen) and the pituitary gland (prolactin, luteinizing hormone [LH], thyroid-stimulating hormone [TSH], and follicle-stimulating hormone [FSH]), all of which have an impact on menstruation. He or she may also order an ultrasound of the pelvic area to identify any abnormalities, including polycystic ovaries, or an MRI or CT scan of the head to see if the pituitary or hypothalamus is causing the amenorrhea. Other tests that are sometimes ordered include thyroid function, hysteroscopy (to visually inspect the inside of the uterus), and saline infusion sonography or hysterosalpingogram, both of which allow the clinician to examine the uterus.

PREVENTION AND TREATMENT

Ways to prevent and treat amenorrhea often coincide. Eating a balanced diet, for example, can both prevent amenorrhea and help restart the menstrual cycle in women who have nutritional deficiencies or who have been dieting excessively. Excessive vigorous exercise (e.g., regular long-distance running or gymnastics) may cause your periods to stop, while a moderate exercise program may help restore them. Amenorrhea caused by excessive stress may be resolved if you adopt ways to effectively manage stress.

If excess secretion of prolactin (hyperprolactinemia) is causing amenorrhea, then medications such as bromocriptine or pergolide may be used to restore function to the ovaries. If ovary function cannot be restored, hormone replacement therapy may be needed to resolve estrogen deficiency and help maintain bone density. Women who need their estrogen deficiency resolved but who do not want to become pregnant may be prescribed oral contraceptives.

A natural supplement approach to amenorrhea can include gamma-linolenic acid (GLA), an essential fatty acid that comes mainly from plant-based oils. Linoleic acid, which is found in cooking oils, is converted into GLA in the body. GLA supplements are available as borage oil, black currant seed oil, and evening primrose oil. These essential fatty acids help reduce inflammation and support hormone production. Some experts recommend taking 1,000 to 1,500 mg one or two times daily.

OTHER HELPFUL INFORMATION

Although premature cessation of your menstrual cycle has an upside (who misses tampons, pads, and cramps?), the downside is the potential loss in bone density and the accompanying increased risk of osteoporosis if you experience amenorrhea for more than three to four months. To help prevent damage to your bone health, talk to your health care provider about correcting the lack of periods and make sure you get adequate calcium, vitamin D, and magnesium through diet and supplements.

READ MORE ABOUT IT

American Society for Reproductive Medicine, 1209 Montgomery Highway, Birmingham, AL 35216-2809; 205-978-5000; www.asrm.org.

ICON Health Publications. *Amenorrhea: A Medical Dictionary, Bibliography and Annotated Research Guide to Internet References.* ICON Health Publications, 2004.

Lachowsky M, Winaver D. Psychogenic amenorrhea. *Gynecol Obstet Fertil* 2007 Jan; 35(1): 45–48.

BACTERIAL VAGINOSIS

Bacterial vaginosis is the most common vaginal condition experienced by women of childbearing age. It is not an infection but rather an imbalance of the bacteria that live in the vagina in which there is an increase in the number of "bad" bacteria as compared with the "good" bacteria. This imbalance is often but not always accompanied by vaginal odor, pain, itching, burning, and a vaginal discharge. In fact, many women who have bacterial vaginosis are not aware they have the condition. It is difficult to say how many women have bacterial vaginosis at any one time, largely because about half of women don't have symptoms, and because the infection keeps coming back after the initial episode has been treated successfully.

CAUSES AND RISK FACTORS
Bacterial vaginosis is caused by a loss of the protective acid-producing bacteria (the "good" bacteria) called lactobacilli in the vagina. These bacteria produce a natural disinfectant called hydrogen peroxide, which combines with chlorine in the cervix to produce yet another chemical that fights against bad bacteria. When lactobacilli numbers decline, there is not enough hydrogen peroxide produced, and the end result is that bacteria, including those that cause bacterial vaginosis (e.g., *Gardnerella vaginalis* and anaerobic bacteria, which require no oxygen) take over. Some studies show that women with

bacterial vaginosis have up to a thousand times more anaerobic bacteria than women without the condition.

What experts are not certain about is what causes the number of lactobacilli to decline. Although bacterial vaginosis is not a sexually transmitted disease, sex does play a role. It may be that some men have semen that kills lactobacilli while others do not. Women who are not sexually active and lesbians also get bacterial vaginosis, so health care professionals know that sexual activity is not the only way to contract this disease.

Women who use an IUD are at greater risk of getting bacterial vaginosis (20 percent) than those who use other methods of birth control (6 percent). Routine douching is also associated with a greater risk for the disease.

DIAGNOSIS

Your doctor can diagnose bacterial vaginosis by your signs and symptoms and by taking a sample of fluid from your vagina for testing while doing a pelvic examination. To make the diagnosis, your clinician is looking for several factors, including:

- Clue cells (cells from the wall of the vagina), which are unique to bacterial vaginosis

- Vaginal pH value greater than 4.5, which is an indication because when the pH-lowering lactobacilli are not present, pH levels rise

- A white or gray-white vaginal discharge that sticks to the vaginal walls

- A positive whiff test, which is an indication because of the smell of the proteins produced by the anaerobic bacteria

PREVENTION AND TREATMENT

Although bacterial vaginosis is not considered to be a sexually transmitted disease (in fact, infected women's sexual partners do not need to be treated), it can be transmitted via sexual activity. Therefore one way to prevent bacterial vaginosis is to abstain from sex. Another is to have a sexual relationship with one partner and remain faithful to each other. If you have sex outside of a monogamous relationship, always use condoms. Other preventive measures include having regular pelvic exams and not douching. If you do get bacterial vaginosis, you should finish the entire course of medication, even if you feel better before you complete it.

Bacterial vaginosis is treated with antibiotics, most often either clindamycin or metronidazole. Both drugs are available as pills or in vaginal forms (gel or cream). The problem with these drugs is that neither one can eliminate bacterial vaginosis. In fact, the condition often returns and needs to be treated again. That's because researchers have yet to find a way to successfully maintain healthy levels of lactobacilli in the vagina (but see "Self-Help and Complementary Care"). Twenty-five percent of women will have a recurrence within four to six weeks of treatment, and up to 80 percent of women who have had bacterial vaginosis will get another episode within a year of treatment.

SELF-HELP AND COMPLEMENTARY CARE
Some studies show that use of probiotics—"good" bacteria such as *Lactobacillus acidophilus, L. rhamnosus,* and *L. fermentum*—can restore lactobacilli levels in the vagina. Use of a probiotic supplement may be used both to prevent bacterial vaginosis, especially recurrence, and as a treatment strategy.

OTHER HELPFUL INFORMATION
If you are pregnant and have·symptoms of bacterial vaginosis or if you have had a premature delivery or a low-birth-weight baby in the past, you should be tested for bacterial vaginosis and be treated if you have it. The same antibiotics can be used for both pregnant and nonpregnant women, although the amount of medication you take if you are pregnant may differ from the amount you would be prescribed if you were not pregnant.

READ MORE ABOUT IT

Falagas ME et al. Probiotics for the treatment of women with bacterial vaginosis. *Clin Microbiol Infect* 2007 Jul; 13(7): 657–64.

Reid G et al. Nucleic acid-based diagnosis of bacterial vaginosis and improved management using probiotics lactobacilli. *J Med Food* 2004 Jun 1; 7(2): 223–28.

Romanik MK et al. The bacterial vaginosis—treatment problems. *Wiad Lek* 2007; 60(1–2): 64–67.

BREAST CANCER

"You've got breast cancer" are among the most frightening words any woman can hear, yet when this disease is caught early, those fears can often be defused. In fact, the American Cancer Society reported in 2007 that U.S. breast cancer deaths declined by 2.2 percent per year from 1990 to 2004, partly due to earlier detection and treatment advances. These statistics are encouraging, but we can do more.

Breast cancer is a disease that develops in the breast tissue, usually in the ducts (tubes that transport milk to the nipple) and lobules (glands that produce milk), depending on the type of cancer (see "Types of Breast Cancer"). Early breast cancer usually does not cause any pain or other symptoms. However, if you notice any change in how your breast(s) or nipple(s) look or feel (e.g., a change in the shape or size, red or swollen areas, scaly or tender nipple or areola, a lump or thickening in or near the breast or under the arm, discharge from the nipple), you should see your health care professional as soon as possible. Inflammatory breast cancer, which occurs in less than 2 percent of all cases of invasive breast cancer, is unique because it does not produce a lump or mass. Instead, inflammatory cells attack the skin and lymph vessels and cause the breast to become red, warm, and swollen, and the skin of the breast may look like the peel of an orange.

The National Cancer Institute estimates that 182,460 new

cases of breast cancer will have developed in the United States in 2008 and that 40,480 women will die of the disease. Most cases of breast cancer occur in women older than sixty.

TYPES OF BREAST CANCER

Breast cancer is categorized according to whether it is invasive or noninvasive, as well as to the part of the breast that it affects.

- **Invasive ductal carcinoma** (IDC) is the most common type of breast cancer, accounting for 80 percent of invasive breast cancers. IDC begins in a duct and then invades the fatty tissue of the breast, after which it may spread to other parts of the body (metastasize).

- **Invasive lobular carcinoma** (ILC) begins to grow in the lobules (milk-producing glands) and can spread to other parts of the body. About 10 percent of invasive breast cancers are ILCs.

- **Ductal carcinoma in situ** (DCIS) is a noninvasive breast cancer and the most common of this type. It represents about 20 percent of all new breast cancer cases and is characterized by cancer cells inside the ducts that have not spread into surrounding tissue.

- **Lobular carcinoma in situ** (LCIS) begins in the lobules and stays within their walls. Women who have this type of cancer have a higher risk of developing an invasive breast cancer.

- **Inflammatory breast cancer** is an aggressive and uncommon type of breast cancer, making up 1 to 6 percent of all breast cancer cases. Rather than a lump or mass in the breast, this type of breast cancer is characterized by swelling, discoloration, warmth, and tenderness of the affected breast.

CAUSES AND RISK FACTORS

The likely causes of breast cancer are closely associated with its risk factors, which we talk about below. That is, breast cancer may be caused by genetic factors (e.g., family history, race, mutations), lifestyle/diet (e.g., high fat intake, lack of exercise, obesity), hormones (e.g., age of first menstruation and menopause), and environment (e.g., exposure to toxins, radiation). With that in mind, consider the following risk factors:

- **Age.** The chance of developing breast cancer increases as women get older. The risk is 1 in 233 for women in their thirties; by age eighty-five, the chance is 1 in 8.

- **Personal history of breast cancer.** If you had breast cancer in one breast, you have an increased risk of developing it in the other breast.

- **Presence of abnormal cells.** If you have certain types of abnormal breast cells (e.g., atypical hyperplasia or lobular carcinoma in situ), you are at increased risk of developing breast cancer.

- **Family history.** Women who have a mother, sister, or daughter with the disease are at increased risk, and the risk is greater if the disease developed in these family members before age forty. Having relatives with both breast and ovarian cancer also increases risk.

- **Race.** Breast cancer affects white women more than Hispanic, Asian, or African American women.

- **Age of first menstruation.** Women who had their first menstrual period before age twelve are at increased risk.

- **Age of menopause.** Women who go through menopause after fifty-five are at increased risk.

- **Gene mutations.** Changes in certain genes, including BRCA1 and BRCA2, increase risk.

- **Giving birth.** Women who have never given birth are at increased risk.

- **Radiation exposure.** Exposure to radiation therapy to the chest before age thirty increases the risk of breast cancer.

- **Dense breast tissue.** Older women who have dense breast tissue are at increased risk.

- **Obesity.** Being overweight or obese after menopause increases risk.

- **Alcohol.** The risk of developing breast cancer increases as intake of alcohol rises.

- **Dietary fat.** A high intake of dietary fat, especially saturated and trans fats, may play a role in breast cancer.

- **Being sedentary.** Lack of physical activity may increase risk of the disease.

DIAGNOSIS

Diagnosis of breast cancer typically goes through stages. If you or your health care provider detects a lump or other abnormality either with screening mammography or physical exam, the next step is usually a referral for a diagnostic mammogram, ultrasound, or other type of imaging procedure. Diagnostic mammography is an X-ray exam of the breasts that involves taking more than the usual two views taken during screening mammography. The goal of diagnostic mammography is to identify the exact size and location of the breast abnormality and to image the lymph nodes and area surrounding it. Often, diagnostic mammography can help show if the abnormality is highly likely to be benign.

If the abnormality appears to be noncancerous, the doctor or radiologist may recommend that you return for a follow-up mammogram in about six months. If, however, the abnormality looks suspicious, your health care provider may order an ultrasonogram or a biopsy. Ultrasonography can indicate whether a mass is solid or filled with fluid (cystic). Generally, cancers are solid and cysts are benign. A biopsy is the only definitive way to identify whether the abnormality is cancerous. Between 65 and 80 percent of breast biopsies uncover a benign condition. If you have breast implants, your physician may order a breast MRI. A ductogram may be ordered if you have experienced abnormal nipple discharge and your health care provider suspects your ducts are involved.

PREVENTION AND TREATMENT
To help prevent breast cancer, look at the risk factors and address those that involve things you can change. If you are inactive, make exercise a part of your daily routine; if you're overweight, lose weight. Because breast cancer risks include many factors you cannot change, you are strongly encouraged to practice regular screening, including breast self-examination, an examination by a health care professional, and routine mammograms based on your age and risk factors (see "Mammography" in Part II). Although you may not be able to prevent the disease, detecting it early and treating it promptly can allow you to stop progression of the disease in its tracks.

Surgery is the main treatment for breast cancer, and the exact procedure that is best for you will depend on your personal wishes, the location, size, and type of tumor, and your overall state of health. One piece of information you and your health care professional will use to make the decision is the *stage* of the tumor (see "Staging of Breast Cancer" in Part III), which is based on the size and location of the tumor, the extent of lymph node involvement, and whether the cancer has metastasized.

Surgical procedures that are offered for women who have breast cancer include lumpectomy and various forms of mastectomy, including radical, modified radical, partial, and simple (see "Mastectomy" in Part II). Depending on the staging of the cancer and the outcome of your surgery, you may also undergo radiation treatment, chemotherapy, biological therapy, hormone therapy, or a combination of these treatments.

A 2008 study found that paclitaxel (Taxol), a derivative of the yew tree, improves survival in women who have breast cancer. This FDA-approved drug has been hailed as one of the most significant advances in chemotherapy (see "Chemotherapy" in Part II) and is also effective in women who have ovarian cancer.

SELF-HELP AND COMPLEMENTARY CARE

Complementary medicine offers women many opportunities to relieve some of the stress, depression, pain, and other side effects associated with breast cancer and its treatment. Many cancer treatment centers have instituted complementary medicine programs that include yoga, acupuncture, meditation, tai chi, hypnosis, guided imagery, massage, and herbal medicine, as well as support groups (see "Read More About It"). Good nutrition is especially important for women who have breast cancer and/or who are undergoing cancer treatment, so consultation with a nutritionist who is knowledgeable about the special nutritional needs of cancer patients is recommended.

OTHER HELPFUL INFORMATION

Researchers are gathering increasing evidence of links between diet and breast cancer. For example:

- A 2005 University of California study found that women treated previously for breast cancer who had the highest plasma carotenoid concentrations had a 40 percent reduced risk of breast cancer recurrence. Carotenoids are plant nutrients found in abundance in fruits and vegetables.

- A 2007 World Cancer Research Fund report says there is convincing evidence that alcohol is a cause of breast cancer.

- The phytoestrogens in soybeans and soy foods act as antiestrogens, which means they may block estrogen from reaching the receptors and thus may protect women from developing breast cancer. This benefit from soy appears to be seen among premenopausal women, who still have naturally high estrogen levels. Among postmenopausal women, however, concentrated soy supplements could add estrogen to the body and thus increase the risk of breast cancer. Therefore, the evidence suggests that soy may benefit premenopausal but not postmenopausal women.

READ MORE ABOUT IT

Link, John. *Breast Cancer Survival Manual: A Step-by-Step Guide for the Woman with Newly Diagnosed Breast Cancer.* 4th ed. Holt Paperbacks, 2007.

Miller, Kenneth D. *Choices in Breast Cancer Treatment: Medical Specialists and Cancer Survivors Tell You What You Need to Know.* Johns Hopkins University Press, 2008.

Sparano JA et al. Weekly paclitaxel in the adjuvant treatment of breast cancer. *N Engl J Med* 2008 Apr 17; 358(16): 1663–71.

BREAST CYSTS

Breast cysts are fluid-filled sacs that typically form when the milk-producing glands enlarge. Unlike breast lumps, many breast cysts are not detectable by physical examination. When they can be felt, they move around freely and are not attached to breast tissue. Often they are microscopic in size, but some can grow to the size of a walnut or larger. Simple cysts are usually oval or round and have smooth edges; complex cysts can be filled with debris.

Breast cysts are most common among women ages thirty to sixty. They can occur in both breasts and form anywhere within them. About 10 percent of women have recurring cysts.

CAUSES AND RISK FACTORS
Exactly why the milk-producing glands enlarge is not known. The most likely cause is hormonal fluctuations, especially premenstrually, and an imbalance between the normal production and absorption of fluids, either during normal menstrual cycles or related to hormone replacement therapy used during postmenopause. A deficiency of gamma-linolenic acid (GLA), an essential fatty acid, may have a role, as may intake of methylxanthines, which are found in coffee, black tea, chocolate, and colas. Some experts say wearing bras every day and at night, and especially bras that have underwires, makes women more likely to develop cysts.

DIAGNOSIS

For many women, the first indication that they may have breast cysts comes when abnormal shadows are seen on their mammogram. The next step is to undergo a breast ultrasound, which is a very sensitive and accurate way (95 percent to 100 percent accuracy) to identify and diagnose breast cysts. In virtually all cases, breast cysts diagnosed by ultrasound are benign; in fact, only about 1 in 1,000 cysts are found to contain a tumor, and even these are not always malignant. By itself, having breast cysts does not increase your risk for breast cancer.

Your health care provider may suggest aspirating the lump (inserting a needle to detect and/or withdraw fluid). This simple technique can confirm that the lump is indeed a cyst; if the lump is solid, the aspirated sample can be analyzed in a laboratory. If your cyst was discovered by ultrasound, aspiration is usually not necessary unless the cyst is causing discomfort or it has abnormal features that indicate it should be explored further.

PREVENTION AND TREATMENT

Because breast cysts are affected by how much fluid you retain, one way to help prevent breast cysts is to limit your salt intake to less than 1,500 mg daily (that's ¾ teaspoon). If that sounds a bit restrictive, reduce your salt intake as much as possible and enjoy some natural diuretics (e.g., artichokes, celery, cucumbers, green tea, parsley, watermelon), which can help reduce fluid retention.

Breast cysts normally do not require treatment unless they are causing you discomfort, in which case aspiration (as noted above) can provide relief. Surgery is rarely necessary.

SELF-HELP AND COMPLEMENTARY CARE

Various nutritional supplements may be most helpful in relieving any pain and discomfort associated with breast cysts and even in helping to prevent them. Here are some options to consider:

- **Vitamin B$_6$** may reduce the swelling and size of breast cysts that are associated with premenstrual syndrome. A suggested dose is 150 mg daily. Also take a vitamin B complex supplement to help keep your B vitamins in balance.

- **Evening primrose oil** may help prevent development of breast cysts. A suggested dose is two 500 mg capsules three times daily.

- **Vitamin C, beta-carotene, and zinc** may reduce symptoms of breast cysts. Suggested daily doses are 30,000 IU beta-carotene (in divided doses), 1,000 mg of vitamin C with bioflavonoids (one to three times daily), and 15 mg of zinc along with 3 mg of copper.

- **The herb chasteberry** (10 drops of tincture in water each morning in the second half of your menstrual cycle) can help balance hormonal function. Its impact is even greater when it is taken along with evening primrose oil and vitamin B$_6$.

OTHER HELPFUL INFORMATION

Women often wonder what would happen if they just left their breast cysts alone. Breast cysts seem to have a life of their own: some disappear completely between annual examinations, while others fluctuate in size but linger on. If you have cystic breasts, your health care provider will likely recommend that you have an ultrasound to get a complete evaluation—and for your own peace of mind.

READ MORE ABOUT IT

ICON Health Publications. *Breast Cysts: A Medical Dictionary, Bibliography and Annotated Research Guide to Internet References.* ICON Health Publications, 2004.

Johnson, Ben, and Kathleen Barnes. *The Secret of Health: Breast Wisdom.* Morgan James Publishing, 2008.

Breast Lumps. See "Breast Cancer," "Breast Cysts," "Fibrocystic Breast Changes"; also "A Closer Look at Breast Lumps" in Part III.

CERVICAL CANCER

Cervical cancer accounts for about 6 percent of all the cancers that affect women. The cervix is the organ that connects the body of the uterus to the vagina. The part of the cervix closest to the uterus is called the endocervix; the part next to the vagina is called the exocervix. These two parts meet in the transformation zone, the zone where most cervical cancers develop. According to the American Cancer Society, in 2008 cervical cancer will have developed in 11,070 women, and 3,870 women will die of the disease.

The two main types of cervical cancer are squamous cell carcinoma (80 to 90 percent of all cervical cancer) and adenocarcinoma (10 to 20 percent). Squamous cell carcinoma usually begins in the transformation zone and develops from the cells that cover the exocervix. Adenocarcinoma develops from the mucus-producing gland cells of the endocervix. In a small number of cases, both types of cancer develop.

CAUSES AND RISK FACTORS

Cervical cancers start from cells that have precancerous changes (also known as precancers or cervical dysplasia), but not all women with these cellular changes eventually develop cancer. In fact, the good news is that precancerous cells disappear without treatment for most women.

Cervical dysplasia is caused primarily by the human papillomavirus (HPV), a general term for more than a hundred related viruses. HPV is also the most important risk factor for cervical cancer. About two-thirds of all cervical cancers are caused by HPV 16 and HPV 18. HPV can be spread during vaginal, anal, and oral sex.

If you smoke, you are twice as likely as a nonsmoker to get cervical cancer. Your risk is also greater if you have human immunodeficiency virus (HIV), a history of or current chlamydia infection, or a diet low in fruits and vegetables. Other risk factors include being overweight, giving birth to seven or more children, a history of many sexual partners, and taking oral contraceptives for five years or longer.

DIAGNOSIS

Cervical cancer is typically a slow-growing disease that often does not have symptoms. However, if you do have symptoms (e.g., pelvic pain, pain during intercourse, abnormal vaginal discharge, vaginal bleeding) or if your Pap test results (see "Pap Smear" in Part II) indicate the presence of precancerous or cancer cells, your health care provider will suggest other procedures to make a diagnosis. These include:

- **Biopsy.** A biopsy involves the removal of tissue to look for precancerous or cancerous cells. Your doctor may recommend any of the following types of biopsies, depending on your specific situation. Each of these procedures is discussed in more detail in Part II.

  - **Conization.** Also known as a cone biopsy, the doctor removes a cone-shaped tissue sample.

  - **Endocervical curettage.** A small instrument is used to scrape a small tissue sample from the cervix.

  - **LEEP (loop electrosurgical excision procedure).** A wire loop is used to collect the sample.

  - **Punch biopsy.** A hollow device is used to collect several small samples.

- **Colposcopy.** A procedure that allows the doctor to look at the cervix using a magnifying lens and light.

PREVENTION AND TREATMENT

Routine screening using the Pap test can prevent cervical cancer from developing nearly 100 percent of the time. As of June 2006, another preventive measure available to females ages nine to twenty-six years is the HPV vaccine, which protects against the four HPV types that together cause 70 percent of cervical cancers and 90 percent of genital warts. The vaccine is given over a six-month period in a series of three injections.

Even though most precancerous changes do not develop into cervical cancer, experts generally agree that all precancers should be treated. The treatment approach depends on the stage of the cancer, size of the tumor, your desire to have children, and your age. The prognosis also depends on the stage of cancer, type of cervical cancer, and the tumor size.

The three main types of medical treatment for cervical cancer include chemotherapy, radiation therapy, and surgery. Several surgical options are available, including bilateral salpingo-oophorectomy, conization, cryosurgery, hysterectomy, laser surgery, and LEEP (see Part II for details on some of these procedures).

SELF-HELP AND COMPLEMENTARY CARE

Various home-care and complementary therapies can help relieve the physical and emotional pain, discomfort, and stress associated with cervical cancer. Scores of cancer centers have programs that focus on mind-body medicine—guided imagery, meditation, yoga, deep breathing therapy, tai chi, acupuncture, massage, and other complementary methods—that can help women who have cervical cancer (see Appendix).

OTHER HELPFUL INFORMATION

Here is yet one more reason to eat your fruits and veggies. A 2008 study out of the University at Buffalo that compared women who had cervical cancer with those who did not found that women who had a high intake of plant-based nutrients (e.g., fiber, alpha- and beta-carotene, folate, lutein, and vitamins A, C, and E) had a 40 to 60 percent reduced risk of developing cervical cancer compared with women who ate few fruits and veggies. This finding is similar to results of other studies of the impact of plant-based foods on bladder cancer, breast cancer, stomach cancer, and prostate cancer.

READ MORE ABOUT IT

Dizon, Don S., Paul DiSilvestro, and Michael Krychman. *100 Questions & Answers About Cervical Cancer.* Jones & Bartlett Publishers, 2008.

Ghosh C et al. Dietary intakes of selected nutrients and food groups and risk of cervical cancer. *Nutr Cancer* 2008 May–Jun; 60(3): 331–41.

Spencer, Juliet. *Cervical Cancer.* Chelsea House, 2007.

CHLAMYDIA

Chlamydia is the most often reported bacterial sexually transmitted disease in the United States. Officials with the Centers for Disease Control and Prevention (CDC) believe, however, that the more than 1 million cases reported each year represent only a fraction of the real number of infections that occur. That's because chlamaydia often does not cause symptoms; indeed, 75 percent of women who develop chlamydia have no symptoms. Thus most people who have the disease do not get tested, and among those who are treated for symptoms, many do not get tested to determine a diagnosis. These circumstances have led the CDC to estimate that at least 2.8 million people contract chlamydia each year.

CAUSES AND RISK FACTORS
Chlamydia is caused by the bacteria *Chlamydia trachomatis,* which is transmitted through sexual contact (oral, vaginal, or anal) with an infected person. The risk factors for chlamydia are unsafe sex practices, which include failure to use a condom, sexual activity with infected individuals, and having multiple sex partners.

DIAGNOSIS
Chlamydia and gonorrhea have similar symptoms (abnormal vaginal discharge, burning sensation when urinating) and can have similar complications if not treated. However, treatment

of these two STDs is different, so a correct diagnosis is important. Chlamydia can be diagnosed using a urine test or evaluation of cell samples collected from the cervix using a swab.

PREVENTION AND TREATMENT
Like other STDs, the best way to prevent chlamydia is to abstain from sex; as alternatives, you can be monogamous with a disease-free partner or practice safe sex and use condoms.

To treat and cure chlamydia, a single dose of azithromycin or a seven-day course of doxycycline is the most commonly used approach if you are not pregnant. Your doctor can prescribe other antibiotics if you are pregnant. During treatment, you and your sex partner(s) should not have sex. If your symptoms do not disappear within one to two weeks after you finish treatment, both you and your partner should see a doctor. Three to four months after treatment, it is best to get a follow-up test to make sure the infection has been eliminated.

If chlamydia is left untreated, it can cause serious reproductive problems, which, like the disease itself, may be asymptomatic. If the chlamydia bacteria spread to the uterus, fallopian tubes, and ovaries, it can cause pelvic inflammatory disease, which can then lead to other serious complications (see "Pelvic Inflammatory Disease"). Untreated chlamydial infections can also cause bladder inflammation and make you more susceptible to HIV.

SELF-HELP AND COMPLEMENTARY CARE
Nutritional supplements may speed your recovery and boost your immune system. Friendly bacteria (probiotics), for example, can improve the ability of your immune system to fight bacterial infections such as chlamydia. One billion to 2 billion CFUs (colony-forming units) per day of *Lactobacillus acidophilus* and other beneficial bacteria species is recommended. Another immune system booster is vitamin C with bioflavonoids, at 1,000 mg daily. The mineral zinc may also help your body resist chlamydia; 30 mg daily, along with 3 mg of copper, is suggested.

OTHER HELPFUL INFORMATION

- Women are often reinfected with chlamydia because their sex partners do not get treated. Reinfections place women at great risk for complications, including infertility.

- Infected mothers can pass the disease to their infants during childbirth. Newborns exposed to chlamydia can get eye infections (conjunctivitis) or pneumonia.

READ MORE ABOUT IT

ICON Health Publications. *Chlamydia Trachomatis—A Medical Dictionary, Bibliography and Annotated Research Guide to Internet References.* ICON Health Publications, 2004.

Van der Pol, Barbara, et al. *Chlamydia, The Silent Disease.* Merit Publishing International, 2007.

CHRONIC VULVAR PAIN (VULVODYNIA)

If you have been suffering with pain and burning in your pelvic area for months, pain that makes it impossible to have sex and uncomfortable to sit, then you may have vulvodynia (the term means "painful vulva"). Characteristics of vulvodynia include itching, throbbing, burning, or tenderness of the vulva, which may include the labia, the opening of the vagina, and the vestibular glands (two glands on either side of the vaginal opening). The pain and discomfort can range from mild to severe and linger for hours or days, then disappear only to come back unexpectedly.

The official definition of vulvodynia is unexplained vulvar pain that persists for three months or longer. Vulvodynia is known by many different names, including vulvar pain syndrome, focal vulvitis, vestibular adenitis, vulvar vestibulitis, and chronic vulvar pain. According to a Harvard study funded by the National Institutes of Health, nearly 16 percent of women in the United States suffer from vulvodynia at some time in their lives, and more than 90 percent say they have had ongoing pain for many years. Therefore, approximately 6 million women currently have this condition, with the greatest number being between the ages of eighteen and twenty-five and the least number being older than thirty-five. Experts believe vulvodynia is probably underreported, partly because often there are no visible signs of the disease and partly because women are embarrassed to talk about it with their physicians.

CAUSES AND RISK FACTORS
The causes of vulvodynia are a mystery, but experts believe some contributing factors include:

- A history of vaginal infections (many women who suffer with vulvodynia have been treated for recurrent vaginitis or vaginal yeast infections)

- Injury or irritation of the nerves that surround the vulva

- Muscle spasms

- Fluctuating estrogen levels that occur with menopause

- Allergies or a hypersensitivity of the skin, especially to substances such as soaps, detergents, powders, sprays, and creams, or to fabrics

DIAGNOSIS
According to a Harvard study conducted in 2003, 60 percent of women consult at least three doctors when seeking a diagnosis, and 40 percent of those still do not have a diagnosis after those three visits. One reason may be that the vulvar tissue may look normal even though you have pain. If the tissue is swabbed with a vinegar solution, it may whiten, and a biopsy may show nonspecific inflammation. Generally, however, vulvodynia is diagnosed when other causes for the pain, such as yeast or bacterial infections, are ruled out.

PREVENTION AND TREATMENT
Without knowing the cause of vulvodynia, experts do not know how to prevent it. Treatment focuses on relieving symptoms. If you have vulvodynia, it is recommended that you try several treatment options at the same time to optimize your chances of relief.

• **Medications.** To reduce chronic pain, many women use tricyclic antidepressants, including amitriptyline, desipramine, and nortriptyline. Some anticonvulsants, such as carbamazepine and gabapentin, may also reduce pain. If itching is a problem, antihistamines, such as hydroxyzine, may be helpful.

• **Physical therapy.** Several approaches can be considered here. You may find that Kegel exercises to strengthen your pelvic floor muscles are helpful (see "Kegel Exercises" in Part II). Other physical therapy techniques that have been useful include massage, transcutaneous electrical nerve stimulation, and therapeutic ultrasound.

• **Biofeedback.** You can learn how to control your pelvic muscles and how to enter a relaxed state as a way to decrease pain sensations. Once you learn the techniques with a biofeedback expert, you can do the exercises at home.

• **Topical estrogen.** For some women, applying estrogen cream reduces pain. Your doctor may also recommend using vaginal estrogen tablets, which you can insert into your vagina once or twice weekly to improve vaginal dryness.

• **Local anesthetics.** Your doctor may recommend using a topical lidocaine ointment, which can provide temporary relief. If you apply it about thirty minutes before sexual intercourse, you can reduce your discomfort, although your partner may also experience some temporary numbness during sexual contact.

• **Trigger point injections.** A steroid medication combined with a numbing agent can be injected into specific points where you feel pain.

SELF-HELP AND COMPLEMENTARY CARE
Although you may not be able to completely eliminate your
symptoms, there are steps you can take to significantly reduce
them and improve your quality of life.

- **Cold compresses.** Place cool/cold compresses directly
  on your external genital area to help reduce pain,
  burning, and itching.

- **Bedtime antihistamine.** Taking an antihistamine at
  bedtime may help reduce itching and help you sleep
  better.

- **Use lubricants.** If you are sexually active, use gentle
  lubricants before sexual intercourse.

- **Keep the air flowing.** Avoid wearing tight-fitting
  undergarments that restrict airflow to your genital
  area. Wear cotton underwear and sleep without underwear at night.

- **Avoid hot tubs.** Sitting in a hot tub, for recreational or
  bathing purposes, may make your symptoms worse.

- **Go white.** Use only white, unbleached toilet paper
  and 100 percent cotton sanitary products.

- **Don't overwash.** Washing or scrubbing your genital
  area too often or too hard will increase irritation. Use
  plain water to gently clean your vulva and pat it dry.

READ MORE ABOUT IT
Glazer, Howard I., and Gae Rodke. *The Vulvodynia Survival
Guide: How to Overcome Painful Vaginal Symptoms and
Enjoy an Active Lifestyle.* New Harbinger Publications, 2002.

Harlow BL, Stewart EG. A population-based assessment of
chronic unexplained vulvar pain: have we underestimated the

prevalence of vulvodynia? *J Am Med Womens Assoc* 2003 Spring; 58(2): 82–88.

Stewart, Elizabeth G., and Paula Spencer. *The V Book: A Doctor's Guide to Complete Vulvovaginal Health.* Bantam, 2002.

Eclampsia. *See* "Preeclampsia."

ECTOPIC PREGNANCY

An ectopic pregnancy (*ectopic* means "out of place") occurs when a fertilized egg implants outside the uterus. In about 98 percent of cases, the pregnancy occurs in the fallopian tubes, which is why ectopic pregnancy is often called "tubal pregnancy." On rare occasions the egg implants in the abdomen, cervix, or ovary. Because none of these areas can support a pregnancy, the organ that contains the growing fetus will eventually burst, resulting in severe bleeding and threatening the life of the mother. The growing tissue may also destroy the organ to which it is attached.

CAUSES AND RISK FACTORS
In the majority of cases, an ectopic pregnancy occurs when a fertilized egg gets stuck in the fallopian tube because the tube is damaged or misshapen. Such pregnancies can occur in women of any age, but the risk is greatest for women who are older than thirty-five. Overall, 2 percent of pregnancies are ectopic.

Besides age, other risk factors for ectopic pregnancy include the following:

- A history of pelvic inflammatory disease

- A history of ectopic pregnancy

- Surgery on a fallopian tube

- Use of fertility drugs or in vitro fertilization

- Pregnancy that occurs while you are using progesterone-only oral contraceptives, an IUD, or the morning-after pill

- Multiple sex partners

- Presence of endometriosis or fibroid tumors

- Cigarette smoking

DIAGNOSIS

Even with today's sophisticated equipment, it is difficult to detect pregnancy less than five weeks after the last menstrual period. Symptoms of ectopic pregnancy are the same as those of early normal pregnancy (e.g., missed periods, tender breasts, nausea, vomiting, frequent urination), which typically appear at six to eight weeks after conception. This similarity makes it difficult to detect an ectopic pregnancy. The first warning signs of an ectopic pregnancy are usually vaginal bleeding or sharp, stabbing pain in the abdomen or pelvis that may be isolated to one side of the pelvis or that comes and goes. Other symptoms may include lower back pain, dizziness, and low blood pressure.

If you go to an emergency department with early warning signs, you will likely be given a urine pregnancy test unless you already know you are pregnant. Once it's determined that you are pregnant, you'll be given a quantitative human chorionic gonadotropin (hCG) test, which measures levels of this hormone, which is produced by the placenta. Lower levels than expected may indicate an ectopic pregnancy. The next step is to get an ultrasound examination: a transvaginal ultrasound is usually more useful than a pelvic ultrasound, but even the transvaginal procedure may not detect an ectopic pregnancy if you are only a few weeks pregnant. If an ultra-sound and a pelvic exam fail to detect anything abnormal, your doctor will likely ask you to return to the hospital or office every two to three days to have your hCG levels retested and to undergo another ultrasound until a pregnancy can be seen.

PREVENTION AND TREATMENT

You cannot prevent an ectopic pregnancy, but you can reduce certain risk factors. For example, practice safe sex to prevent contracting a sexually transmitted disease; don't smoke; and limit the number of sexual partners. If you have a history of ectopic pregnancy, consult your health care provider before you become pregnant again.

Some ectopic pregnancies resolve themselves; however, because they pose a serious risk of rupture, bleeding, and even death, most health care professionals recommend either drug or surgical intervention as soon as possible. An injection of methotrexate can stop the growth of the embryo in an early pregnancy (less than six weeks), although it usually takes several weeks for the pregnancy to completely resolve. An ectopic pregnancy that is further along should be treated surgically. Unless it is an emergency situation, the embryo can usually be removed using laparoscopy, a minimally invasive surgical procedure (see "Pelvic Laparoscopy" in Part II) that uses tiny incisions and requires minimal recovery time. If the pregnancy is complicated because of the location of the embryo or other factors, a more invasive surgical procedure called a laparotomy may be needed.

Regardless of which treatment approach is used, your doctor will need to take several additional readings of your hCG levels to make sure the ectopic pregnancy has been eliminated.

OTHER HELPFUL INFORMATION

- Once you have had an ectopic pregnancy, your chances of having another are 15 to 20 percent; if you have had a second ectopic pregnancy, your chances of having a third are about 32 percent.

• The chance of having an ectopic pregnancy if you have undergone in vitro fertilization to get pregnant ranges from 2 to 11 percent.

READ MORE ABOUT IT

Bignardi T et al. Is ultrasound the new gold standard for the diagnosis of ectopic pregnancy? *Semin Ultrasound CT MR* 2008 Apr; 29(2): 114–20.

Dengfeng W et al. Chinese herbal medicines in the treatment of ectopic pregnancy. *Cochrane Database Syst Rev* 2007 Oct 17; (4):CD006224.

Gajewska M et al. Laparoscopic management of ectopic pregnancy. *Neuro Endocrinol Lett* 2008 Apr; 29(2): 267–71.

Levine D. Ectopic pregnancy. *Radology* 2007 Nov; 245(2):385–97.

ENDOMETRIAL CANCER

Each year, about 40,000 women are diagnosed with endometrial cancer, a disease that involves the lining of the uterus, or endometrium. For this reason it is often referred to as uterine cancer, although in about 5 percent of cases other types of cells in the uterus become cancerous. Endometrial cancer is the most common gynecologic cancer and the fourth most common cancer found in women (behind breast, lung, and colon cancer), and typically strikes postmenopausal women, although a small percentage of cases affect women younger than forty.

The most common sign of endometrial cancer is abnormal vaginal bleeding. A white, pink, or watery discharge from the vagina, pain during intercourse, weight loss, and pelvic pain also are indications of endometrial cancer. The good thing about endometrial cancer is that it generally grows slowly and rarely reaches an advanced stage before signs and symptoms are apparent.

CAUSES AND RISK FACTORS

Experts are not certain why endometrial cells mutate and become cancerous, but they believe estrogen plays a major role. Some researchers are also looking into how changes in genes may contribute to the disease.

Risk factors for endometrial cancer revolve around estrogen levels. When the balance between progesterone and estrogen shifts toward the latter, the endometrium thickens, which increases the risk of cancer. Therefore, factors that elevate estrogen levels are risk factors for endometrial cancer and include the following:

- **The more years you menstruate.** This translates into more exposure to estrogen and a greater risk. A good example is a woman who started menstruation before age twelve and who continued to menstruate into her fifties.

- **Never having been pregnant.** Although estrogen levels are high during pregnancy, the accompanying high progesterone levels appear to protect against any detrimental effects of estrogen.

- **Obesity.** Fat tissue can elevate your estrogen levels by changing some hormones into estrogen.

- **Type 2 diabetes.** Some research suggests that having type 2 diabetes increases a woman's risk of endometrial cancer. Part of the reason may be that obesity is common among women who have diabetes, yet the risk of endometrial cancer is also higher among diabetic women who are not overweight.

- **Tamoxifen.** One in every 500 women who take tamoxifen for breast cancer will develop endometrial cancer. If you are using this hormone, you should have an annual pelvic exam to screen for any abnormalities.

- **Estrogen replacement therapy.** Estrogen stimulates growth of the endometrium and thus increases cancer risk, while combination replacement therapy (progesterone and estrogen) can help prevent endometrial cancer. This combination, however, carries other health risks (see "Hormone Replacement Therapy" in Part II).

DIAGNOSIS
Your gynecologist or other health care professional will do a physical and pelvic examination and feel for any abnormalities in the uterus. If any problems are detected, your doctor may want to get cell samples from inside your uterus (an endometrial biopsy) or perform a transvaginal ultrasound, which creates a video image of the inside of the uterus (see "Biopsy" and "Ultrasound" in Part II). If an adequate tissue sample can't be taken or if the biopsy suggests cancer, a dilatation and curettage (D & C) may be necessary to scrape a sample from the lining of your uterus (see "Dilatation and Curettage" in Part II). If endometrial cancer is found, more tests will be needed to determine if the cancer has spread, which may include a computerized tomography scan, a chest X-ray, and a blood test that measures CA-125, a substance that is released by some endometrial and ovarian cancers.

PREVENTION AND TREATMENT
Most cases of endometrial cancer can't be prevented, but you can reduce your risk of developing the disease if you:

- **Maintain a healthy body weight.** The presence of excess body fat promotes estrogen production, which increases your risk of endometrial cancer.

- **Have a history of oral contraceptive use.** The use of birth control pills reduces your risk of developing endometrial cancer, even for as long as a decade after you stop taking them.

- **Take hormone replacement therapy (HRT).** Combination hormone therapy reduces your risk of endometrial cancer, but bear in mind that the progestin/estrogen combo can cause other serious side effects. Talk with your doctor to decide whether HRT is best for you.

If you get a diagnosis of endometrial cancer, the most common treatment is surgery—either removal of the uterus or the uterus along with the fallopian tubes and ovaries (see "Hysterectomy" in Part II). If the cancer is aggressive and/or it has spread to other parts of the body, additional treatments may be required, including chemotherapy, radiation, and hormone therapy.

SELF-HELP AND COMPLEMENTARY CARE
Many cancer treatment centers now offer complementary therapies to help reduce the stress, pain, and uncertainty often associated with cancer. Whether you take advantage of these therapies at such centers or you explore them on your own or with friends or self-help groups, you should know that studies show that practices such as yoga, meditation, tai chi, relaxation and imagery training, and massage can be most helpful for women who have cancer.

READ MORE ABOUT IT
ICON Health Publications. *Endometrial Cancer: A Medical Dictionary, Bibliography and Annotated Research Guide to Internet References.* ICON Health Publications, 2004.

PM Medical Health News. *21st Century Complete Medical Guide to Uterine Cancer (Endometrial Cancer, Cancer of the Uterus).* PM Medical Health News, 2002. CD-ROM.

ENDOMETRIAL POLYPS

Endometrial polyps are an overgrowth of endometrial tissue that develop inside the uterus and can grow into and through the cervix, and even extend into the vagina. Not all women who have endometrial polyps experience symptoms, but when they do, they may have cramping pain, highly irregular periods, bleeding between periods or after menopause, and infertility. Endometrial polyps are most likely to occur in women who are younger than fifty and may appear as a single polyp or as several together. Although endometrial polyps can be bothersome, the vast majority of them are benign.

CAUSES AND RISK FACTORS
You are more likely to develop endometrial polyps if you have high blood pressure, if you have had cervical polyps, if you are obese, or if you take tamoxifen (which is for breast cancer). However, experts are uncertain about what causes endometrial polyps. Evidence points to a role for hormones, especially estrogen.

DIAGNOSIS
If you have signs and/or symptoms of endometrial polyps, a common diagnostic tool is transvaginal ultrasound, which uses sound waves to explore the inside of the uterus (see "Ultrasound" in Part II). A hysteroscopy, which is a combination diagnostic tool and treatment that involves inserting a thin,

flexible lighted telescope into the uterus, is another option. Another combination diagnostic/treatment method is curettage, which allows practitioners to both collect specimens and remove polyps with the same instrument. Yet another treatment approach is the use of medication, specifically progestins and gonadotropin-releasing hormone agonists, which may relieve symptoms and shrink a uterine polyp. Medications are not a permanent solution, however, as symptoms typically return once you stop treatment.

PREVENTION AND TREATMENT

Experts have not identified a way to prevent endometrial polyps. In fact, once a polyp has been removed, it may recur. Some small, asymptomatic polyps disappear on their own without treatment, while others can be treated with hormonal medications to help shrink them and thus reduce symptoms. Treatment is usually not necessary unless you are at risk of endometrial cancer or your symptoms are severe. In such cases, surgery is a common option and may include either excision (removal) of the polyps or hysterectomy if the polyps contain cancerous cells (see "Hysterectomy" in Part II).

SELF-HELP AND COMPLEMENTARY CARE

According to traditional Chinese medicine, polyps can be managed and treated using herbs that strengthen the spleen and kidney and that are drying in nature. If you are interested in exploring complementary treatment with Chinese medicine, we recommend that you consult a Chinese herbal practitioner to receive the appropriate herbs to match your specific condition.

OTHER HELPFUL INFORMATION

It is uncertain whether having endometrial polyps leads to infertility, but at least one study found that infertile women who had their polyps removed had a much higher pregnancy rate after intrauterine insemination than did women with polyps who underwent intrauterine insemination alone. Having endometrial polyps may also increase your risk of miscarriage if you plan to undergo in vitro fertilization.

READ MORE ABOUT IT

Hileeto D et al. Age-dependent association of endometrial polyps with increased risk of cancer involvement. *World J Surg Oncol* 2005 3:8.

Taylor E, Gomel V. The uterus and fertility. *Fertil Steril* 2008 Jan; 89(1): 1–16.

.

ENDOMETRIOSIS

Endometriosis is a chronic, painful, and often debilitating condition that affects more than 5.5 million females ages eight to eighty in the United States and Canada, although it most often affects women during their reproductive years. The disease involves the growth of cells that typically form the inside of the uterus (the endometrial cells), but which grow on sites outside the uterus, forming what are called endometriosis implants. The implants are most often found on the ovaries, the fallopian tubes, on the outer surfaces of the uterus or intestines, and on the lining of the pelvic cavity. Rarely, they occur on the liver, outside the pelvis, or around the lung or brain.

Although endometriosis implants are typically benign, they do pose a risk: according to the National Cancer Institute and the National Institutes of Health, endometriosis places women at greater risk for various cancers and autoimmune diseases, including fibromyalgia, chronic fatigue syndrome, rheumatoid arthritis, multiple sclerosis, systemic lupus erythematosus, and eczema. They also can cause significant pelvic pain, cramping with intercourse, and infertility. Occasionally some women also experience abdominal pain, diarrhea, constipation, low back pain, or bloody urine.

CAUSES AND RISK FACTORS

The cause of endometriosis is unknown, although experts have a few theories. One is that during menstruation, some of the menstrual tissue makes its way into the fallopian tubes and then implants in the abdomen and grows. Another suggests that endometriosis is an immune-system response to endometrial cells that enter the abdomen, and there is also interest in the possible role of environmental toxins, such as dioxin (PCBs), found in pesticides and herbicides. A genetic abnormality that causes endometrial cells to grow outside the uterus during fetal development is yet another possibility. Whatever the cause may be, it appears that there are no specific risk factors for the disease.

DIAGNOSIS

Discovery of endometriosis usually begins with a medical history review and pelvic examination. During the examination, the physician feels and looks for enlarged ovaries, lesions on the vagina, nodules, or pain and/or tenderness in the pelvic area. If the findings from these efforts raise suspicions, your physician may do a laparoscopy, which will allow him or her to determine the extent of the disease and how to best treat it (see "Pelvic Laparoscopy" in Part II). Many women elect not to have the laparoscopy done if their symptoms are mild to moderate, choosing instead to try treatment. If treatment is not successful (see "Prevention and Treatment"), laparoscopy may be helpful in getting a better picture of the problem.

Some health care professionals use biochemical markers to make a diagnosis. Many women with endometriosis, for example, have high levels of a substance called CA-125, or a protein known as PP14. The use of tests for these biochemical markers may soon replace the need for laparoscopy to diagnose endometriosis.

PREVENTION AND TREATMENT

Because the exact cause of endometriosis is unknown, there are no definitive ways to prevent this disease. However, there are several treatment approaches you can take, depending on how severe your symptoms are and whether you plan to get pregnant.

To treat pain, anti-inflammatory drugs (e.g., ibuprofen,

naproxen) or birth control hormones may be sufficient. Anti-inflammatories reduce inflammation, pain, and bleeding, while birth control hormones help shrink endometrial tissue and may also prevent endometriosis from getting worse. If your pain is severe or does not respond well to these methods, you may try a stronger hormone therapy such as progestin, gonadotropin-releasing hormone agonist (GnRH-a), or an aromatase inhibitor (e.g., anastrozole, letrozole).

If hormone therapy does not offer relief or if you have endometrial growths that are affecting other organs, you may need to have the growths surgically removed. In most cases, this can be done through laparoscopy and provides pain relief for a year or two in most women (see "Pelvic Laparoscopy" in Part II), but no relief for about 20 percent of women. Endometriosis usually returns after several years.

In severe cases, another option is removal of the uterus and ovaries (see "Hysterectomy" in Part II). Even this dramatic step fails to bring relief to up to 15 percent of women.

SELF-HELP AND COMPLEMENTARY CARE

What you eat can impact your risk of endometriosis and your experience with it. For example, studies show that fresh fruits and vegetables are associated with a reduced risk of endometriosis, while eating red meat and ham increase your risk. Plant chemicals (phytonutrients) called indoles, which are found in broccoli, cauliflower, kale, and other cruciferous vegetables, seem to improve estrogen metabolism, which may reduce risk and symptoms. Omega-3 fatty acids found in fish oils have also been found to decrease inflammation and may slow the growth of endometrial tissue. Certain fish, such as salmon, herring, and sardines, as well as fish oil supplements, provide this nutrient.

Another self-help approach is a contrast sitz bath. Prepare two basins or tubs in which you can sit comfortably. Fill one with hot water and the other with cool to cold. Sit in the hot water for three minutes, then in the cooler water for one minute. Repeat this cycle three more times. Do not use a sitz bath during menstruation.

OTHER HELPFUL INFORMATION

Endometriosis is a cause of infertility, but one that is not completely understood. Some experts believe endometriosis affects fertility by producing hormones that have a negative impact on ovulation, egg fertilization, or implantation of the embryo in the uterus. Others say endometriosis may cause scar tissue that hinders transportation of the eggs from the ovaries. If you have endometriosis and are planning pregnancy (or if you are having difficulty getting pregnant), talk to your doctor about the possible impact of endometriosis on your fertility.

READ MORE ABOUT IT

Morris, Kerry-Ann. *Living Well with Endometriosis: What Your Doctor Doesn't Tell You . . . That You Need to Know.* Collins, 2006.

Panay N. Advances in the medical management of endometriosis. *BJOG* 2008 Jun; 115(7): 814–17.

Worwood, Valerie Ann, and Julia Stonehouse. *The Endometriosis Natural Treatment Program: A Complete Self-Help Plan for Improving Health and Well-Being.* New World Library, 2007.

ENDOMETRIOSIS OF THE UTERUS (ADENOMYOSIS)

Adenomyosis is a condition in which the endometrium—the tissue that normally lines the uterus—grows inside the walls of the uterus, causing the walls to harden. This condition is sometimes referred to as "endometriosis of the uterus," yet it is different from endometriosis, even though women who have adenomyosis often have both conditions (see "Endometriosis"). Women most affected by adenomyosis are those in their mid- to upper forties.

Adenomyosis can be quite painful, but not all women experience symptoms of this otherwise harmless disorder. When symptoms occur, they can include:

- Prolonged or heavy menstrual flow

- Passing blood clots during menstruation

- Severe cramping or sharp pelvic pain during menstruation

- Bleeding between periods

- Pain during intercourse

- Enlarged uterus (double to triple its normal size), often accompanied by a tender, enlarged lower abdomen

CAUSES AND RISK FACTORS

The cause of adenomyosis is unknown. Experts do know, however, that this abnormal tissue growth depends on estrogen. Theories about why the tissue invades the uterine walls include the possibility that adenomyosis originates from endometrial tissue that was left there when the female fetus was developing. Some researchers suggest that inflammation of the endometrium after childbirth may cause a break in the cells lining the uterus and allow abnormal growth to begin. Women at greater risk of adenomyosis include those who have undergone a cesarian section, surgical removal of fibroids, or uterine surgery. The condition is also more common among women who have given birth to at least one child.

DIAGNOSIS

Your doctor may strongly suspect adenomyosis based on:

- Your signs and symptoms

- An enlarged uterus, which can be identified during a pelvic exam

- Endovaginal ultrasound (also called transvaginal ultrasound) or magnetic resonance imaging (MRI) of the uterus

Several other uterine diseases cause symptoms similar to those associated with adenomyosis, including fibroid tumors, endometriosis, and endometrial polyps. At one time a definitive diagnosis of adenomyosis could be made only after the uterus was removed (hysterectomy), but today endovaginal ultrasonography or MRI, when done by experienced technicians, can provide accurate diagnostic information.

PREVENTION AND TREATMENT

If you have adenomyosis and you are approaching or are already experiencing menopause, the good news is that this condition typically disappears after menopause. However, if you are not near menopause or you need relief from your symptoms *now,* your health care professionals may suggest the following:

- **Anti-inflammatory drugs** can help, especially if you are near menopause. Use of anti-inflammatory medications (e.g., ibuprofen, naproxen) several days before your period begins and throughout menstruation may provide significant relief.

- **Hormone therapy** may reduce heavy bleeding, cramping, and other pain.

- **Hysterectomy** may be suggested if your pain is severe and menopause is many years away. Removal of the ovaries is not necessary.

- **Hysteroscopic endometrial ablation** (surgical removal of the lining of the uterus) may provide relief if heavy bleeding rather than cramps is the main symptom. This surgery is typically performed as an outpatient procedure.

- **Laser technology** (CO_2, YAG, and argon) is an alternative approach used by some practitioners for women who want to remain fertile. Laser preserves the endometrial cavity but treats the invaded uterine muscle.

SELF-HELP AND COMPLEMENTARY CARE
Studies show that acupuncture and therapeutic massage from a health care professional can provide pain relief. A home remedy is the use of contrast sitz baths. Find two basins that you can sit in comfortably and put hot water in one, cool to cold in the other. Sit in hot water for three minutes, then in cold water for one minute. Repeat this three times to complete one set and do one or two sets each day, three to four days per week. Sitz baths should not be done while you are menstruating.

OTHER HELPFUL INFORMATION

If you undergo endometrial ablation for adenomyosis and you are sexually active but do not want to get pregnant, you should continue to use birth control even though the chance of getting pregnant after this procedure is low.

READ MORE ABOUT IT

Bickerstaff H. The presurgical diagnosis of diffuse adenomyosis. Retrieved on April 27, 2008, from www.obgyn.net/women/women.asp?page=/eago/art04.

Sun YZ, Chen HL. Controlled study on Shu-Mu point combination for treatment of endometriosis. *Zhongguo Zhen Jiu* 2006 Dec; 26(12): 863–65.

Worwood, Valerie Ann, and J. Stonehouse. *The Endometriosis Natural Treatment Program: A Complete Self-Help Plan for Improving Health and Well-Being.* New World Library, 2007.

FIBROADENOMA

A fibroadenoma is a benign breast tumor composed of glandular and fibrous materials. These tumors are found in 10 percent of all women (20 percent of African American women) and most often in young women between the ages of fifteen and thirty. Fibroadenomas are often described as feeling like marbles—round, movable, firm, and slightly rubbery. Another telltale sign of fibroadenomas is that while some breast lumps come and go during the menstrual cycle, fibroadenomas usually do not disappear after your period.

Between 85 and 90 percent of women who have a fibroadenoma have only one, and it typically ranges in size from 1 to 5 cm. Rarely, fibroadenomas can be as big as a plum.

CAUSES AND RISK FACTORS

The cause of fibroadenomas is unknown. Estrogen appears to play a major role, because these growths are common in premenopausal women, they grow large in pregnant women, and they can appear in postmenopausal women who are taking estrogen.

Your risk for developing fibroadenomas is greater if you are younger than thirty-five years old and if you have a history of benign breast lesions. Your risk decreases the longer you use oral contraceptives and the more times you are pregnant.

DIAGNOSIS

Your health care professional will take a complete personal and family medical history and ask questions about the lump if you are the one who discovered it. After he or she does a physical exam, a mammogram or ultrasound may be scheduled or the doctor may order a biopsy—either a fine-needle aspiration, core, incisional, or excisional biopsy (see "Biopsy" in Part II).

PREVENTION AND TREATMENT

Breast fibroadenomas cannot be prevented. They can be discovered early using breast self-examination.

Treatment can vary from a watch-and-wait approach to surgical removal of the lump. Often fibroadenomas in younger women are monitored with self-examination, yearly professional checkups, and mammograms. Removal is usually recommended for women older than thirty and for those whose lumps are painful and/or growing. Although surgical removal using lumpectomy or surgical excision under local or general anesthesia is still used, a more popular and less invasive approach is cryoablation biopsy, which uses local anesthesia and requires no stitches (see "Biopsy" in Part II).

SELF-HELP AND COMPLEMENTARY CARE

Although the jury is still out on alternative ways to treat fibroadenomas, there are anecdotal reports that a high-fiber, low-fat, plant-based diet is helpful. You may also want to consider taking various nutritional supplements daily to help relieve symptoms: 300 mg vitamin C, 400 IU vitamin E, 1 to 2 tablespoons flaxseed oil, and 1,000 mg fish oil.

READ MORE ABOUT IT

Nelson ZC et al. Risk factors for fibroadenoma in a cohort of female textile workers in Shanghai, China. *Am J Epidemiology* 2002 Oct. 1; 156 (7): 599–605.

Smith GE, Burrows P. Ultrasound diagnosis of fibroadenoma—is biopsy always necessary? *Clin Radiol* 2008 May; 63(5): 511–15.

FIBROCYSTIC BREAST CHANGES

Fibrocystic breast change is a very common and benign condition in which one or both breasts are characterized by lumpiness and varying degrees of pain, discomfort, and tenderness. For some women, the condition occurs only for a few days before their menstrual period; for others, the pain and lumpiness are constant. Sixty to 90 percent of women experience some degree of fibrocystic breast changes, and most of those women are between the ages of thirty and fifty.

CAUSES AND RISK FACTORS

Fibrocystic breast changes are associated with hormonal fluctuations, specifically estrogen and progesterone, because these hormones cause breast cells to grow and multiply. Other hormones also play a role; they include prolactin, growth factor, insulin, and thyroid hormone, as well as hormonal products produced by the breast.

Every month, the cyclical hormones of menstruating women stimulate the growth of breast tissue and increase cell metabolism. All this activity may cause breast fullness and fluid retention. When the menstrual cycle is over, many of the stimulated breast cells die as part of a process called programmed cell death, or apoptosis. During apoptosis, enzymes break down the cells and the resulting cell fragments are broken down further. The amount of debris and the degree of inflammation can vary from month to month, and thus so can the severity of the symptoms you may experience.

DIAGNOSIS

The most common symptom of fibrocystic breast changes is breast pain or discomfort, but you can have this condition without symptoms. If you do have discomfort, it may appear as a feeling of fullness in the breasts, a dull, heavy pain, breast tenderness, and/or itchy nipples. Fibrocystic breasts can be diagnosed by touch: you or your health care practitioner can examine your breasts for lumpiness, which is most often found in the upper outer quadrant of the breast. Lumps associated with fibrocystic breast changes usually feel rounded, smooth, rubbery, and mobile. Some may feel like tiny beads.

Some women have extremely fibrocystic breasts, which makes it difficult to examine them and to determine a diagnosis. Mammograms of such women may be difficult to interpret, and in some cases breast ultrasound examinations or even a biopsy may be necessary in order to make a diagnosis of fibrocystic breast changes or breast cancer.

PREVENTION AND TREATMENT

There are many anecdotal reports that reducing intake of dietary fat and caffeine can help prevent or reduce symptoms of fibrocystic breasts. Although there are no scientific studies to back up these claims, both are healthy steps you may want to take.

Treatment of fibrocystic breast changes may be as easy as wearing a more supportive bra or wearing a bra at night (but see "Other Helpful Information") or taking anti-inflammatory medications. Correcting hormonal imbalances using oral contraceptives can be helpful in women who have very irregular menstrual cycles, as it can regulate their cycles and allow the breast tissue to recover more completely.

SELF-HELP AND COMPLEMENTARY CARE

Several vitamins and supplements may help reduce symptoms of fibrocystic breast changes. One is oil of primrose, which contains certain essential fatty acids that may help reduce breast pain. A suggested dose to relieve symptoms is two to eight 500 mg capsules daily: lower doses are effective for breast tenderness, while higher doses help relieve pain and inflammation. Vitamins C (300 mg daily), E (200–600 IU), B_6 (2 mg), and A (5,000 IU) are also recommended.

OTHER HELPFUL INFORMATION
In 1995, a research team published a book in which they claimed that wearing a bra increases the risk of developing fibrocystic breasts and breast cancer. *Dressed to Kill: The Link Between Breast Cancer and Bras* notes that bras can constrict the flow of lymphatic fluid, which helps flush toxins from the breasts and body. The fluids instead can pool and result in fibrocystic changes (benign lumps, pain, and cysts) and create the potential for breast cancer. Although this claim has never been proven, some experts suggest that women not wear a bra at night and that very restrictive bras, such as those with underwires, be avoided when possible.

READ MORE ABOUT IT
Campbell EM et al. Premenstrual symptoms in general practice patients. Prevalence and treatment. *J Reprod Med* 1997 Oct; 42(10): 637–46.

Campbell PF. Relieving endometriosis pain: why is it so tough? *Obstet Gynecol Clin North Am* 2003 Mar; 30(1): 209–20.

Horner LK, Lampe JW. Potential mechanisms of diet therapy for fibrocystic breast conditions show inadequate evidence of effectiveness. *J Am Diet Assoc* 2000 Nov; 100(11): 1368–80.

Singer, Sydney Ross, and Soma Grismaijer. *Dressed to Kill: The Link Between Breast Cancer and Bras.* Avery, 1995.

FIBROIDS

Fibroids (also known as myomas or leiomyomas) are benign growths that can develop in various locations in the uterine wall. Approximately 20 percent of all women older than thirty-five have at least one fibroid, and these growths are found more often in black women than in white women. Fibroids range in size from a pea to a grapefruit and can cause heavy, prolonged menstrual bleeding, a feeling of fullness, and urinary frequency. Most women do not experience pain unless the fibroids press on the rectum or ureters.

Fibroids are classified by their location, which impacts the symptoms they cause and how they can be treated. There are three main types:

- **Intramural or interstitial** fibroids reside deep in the uterine wall. This is the most common type.

- **Subserous** fibroids are found outside the uterus.

- **Submucous** fibroids lie under the uterine lining. These are the least common type. Sometimes these fibroids are connected to the uterine wall by a stalk, in which case they are called pedunculated fibroids.

CAUSES AND RISK FACTORS

The development and growth of fibroids appear to be stimulated by estrogen, and this idea is supported by the fact that these growths typically shrink and disappear after menopause. Risk factors for fibroids include:

- **Age.** Fibroids are more common in women in their thirties and forties through menopause.

- **Family history.** If your mother had fibroids, you have a three times greater risk of developing these growths.

- **Ethnic background.** African American women are more likely to develop fibroids than white women.

- **Animal-based diet.** Eating red meat and ham is associated with a greater risk of fibroids.

- **Obesity.** Being overweight increases your risk for fibroids, and obesity elevates the risk to two to three times greater than average.

DIAGNOSIS

It can be difficult to make a diagnosis based on a pelvic examination because fibroids can feel like an ovarian cyst or be confused with adenomyosis. That's why physicians often resort to laparoscopy to make a diagnosis. A submucous fibroid often must be verified using biopsy or ultrasound.

PREVENTION AND TREATMENT

If you have small fibroids that cause minimal symptoms or larger ones that cause little discomfort, you will likely not need treatment. Intramural and subserous fibroids rarely need treatment unless they grow to be very large or they are pressing on the bowel or bladder. Submucous fibroids usually require treatment because they cause severe menstrual problems.

Surgical removal of fibroids is called myomectomy. Some fibroids can be removed using laparoscopy. Large fibroids may be shrunk using laser or electric needles. Several newer treatment techniques include radiofrequency ablation, which uses radio waves to destroy fibroids; focused ultrasound, which beams high-intensity ultrasound energy at the growth for several hours; and uterine artery embolization, which shrinks fibroids by cutting off their blood supply.

If you are approaching menopause, your doctor may suggest hormonal therapy as an alternative to surgery. Natural, bioidentical progesterone therapy rather than synthetic progestin can help shrink fibroids when used for six months or longer.

SELF-HELP AND COMPLEMENTARY CARE

A University of Arizona study found that traditional Chinese medicine (including acupuncture and herbal formulas), guided imagery, and body work were effective in relieving symptoms of fibroids. Some women say their fibroids have shrunk or dissolved after taking chasteberry (vitex) for as little as two months, although there is little scientific evidence to support these claims. A suggested dose is two 250 mg tablets, 40 drops of extract, or 120 drops tincture daily first thing in the morning. Chasteberry works best for fibroids on the uterus and not in deep tissue.

OTHER HELPFUL INFORMATION

If you have fibroids and are pregnant, the location of the growths may impact your delivery. Fibroids rarely interfere with pregnancy because they usually move out of the pelvis and up into the abdomen, which allows you to have a normal vaginal delivery. If the fibroids remain in the pelvis, however, you may need to have a cesarean section.

READ MORE ABOUT IT

Chiaffarino F et al. Diet and uterine myomas. *Obstet Gynecol* 1999 Sep; 94(3): 395–98.

Mehl-Madrona L. Complementary medicine treatment of uterine fibroids: a pilot study. *Altern Ther Health Med* 2002 Mar–Apr; 8(2): 34–36.

Mukhopadhaya N. Conventional myomectomy. *Best Pract Res Clin Obstet Gynaecol* 2008 Apr 3.

GENITAL HERPES

Genital herpes is a sexually transmitted disease caused by a virus that can stay in the body indefinitely. The infection is more common in women than in men: it affects about 25 percent of women and 12 percent of men. Most people with genital herpes have no or mild signs or symptoms, which may include burning, itching, tingling, or pain around the rectum or genitals, followed by the appearance of red spots and blisters. In some cases, people also experience flulike symptoms, including fever and swollen glands. Women are more likely to develop painful urination, and the warning here is to avoid a urinary tract infection by drinking lots of fluids to dilute your urine.

When the blisters break they leave sores (ulcers) that may take up to four weeks to heal the first time they occur. Subsequent outbreaks of the disease can happen at any time, but they are nearly always less severe and shorter in duration than the first outbreak.

CAUSES AND RISK FACTORS

Genital herpes can be caused by two different herpes simplex viruses: type 1 (HSV-1) or type 2 (HSV-2). Most genital herpes is caused by HSV-2 and is spread through sexual contact—vaginal, anal, and/or oral. The more sexual partners you have had, the greater your risk for genital herpes. Failure to use a condom also increases your risk.

DIAGNOSIS

Because the signs and symptoms associated with HSV-2 can vary greatly, the most accurate ways for health care professionals to make a diagnosis are to do a physical examination during an outbreak and to take a sample from a sore for lab analysis. If there is no outbreak, the infection can be diagnosed using a blood test, although the results are not always accurate.

Another kind of test is the direct fluorescent antibody test, in which a solution containing HSV antibodies and a fluorescent dye is added to a sample taken from a sore. If the virus is in the sample, the antibodies will glow when viewed under a special microscope.

PREVENTION AND TREATMENT

The only sure way to avoid contracting genital herpes is to abstain completely from sexual contact or to be in a mutually monogamous sexual relationship in which both of you have been tested and are free of infection. Properly used, latex condoms can greatly reduce your risk of getting the disease, and they should be used in all situations unless you are in a monogamous relationship. Keep in mind that if you or your sexual partner has genital herpes and has no symptoms, you can still spread the disease.

Although there is no cure for genital herpes, several antiviral medications are available to help reduce the frequency and severity of outbreaks and the chance of transmitting the disease to others. The three main drugs used to treat genital herpes are acyclovir, famciclovir, and valacyclovir. All are available as pills, and acyclovir can be given intravenously for severe infections.

If you have genital herpes and have already been treated with antiviral drugs for your first outbreak, there are two ways you can continue treatment: intermittent therapy, in which you take medication when you feel an outbreak is approaching and then stop the drug once the outbreak has passed, or suppressive therapy, in which you take an antiviral medication every day, with the hope of significantly reducing the frequency and severity of any outbreaks.

SELF-HELP AND COMPLEMENTARY CARE

Honeybees produce a waxy substance called propolis, and an ointment that contains propolis may help herpes sores heal faster. One study showed, for example, that 80 percent of patients who used a propolis ointment had healed sores after ten days, compared with only 47 percent of patients who used acyclovir ointment and 40 percent who used a placebo.

Many people have success using the amino acid L-lysine. At the first sign of an outbreak, the suggested dose is 1,000 mg with each meal, then reduce to 500 mg when your symptoms lessen. This is also the suggested maintenance dose to help prevent outbreaks. While lysine can help prevent outbreaks, another amino acid, arginine, may trigger them, so it is best to avoid foods that are rich in this substance, including chocolate, peanuts, seeds, cereal grains such as oatmeal, raisins, and carob.

Other supplements that may help reduce recurrence of herpes outbreaks include zinc (22.5 mg daily), vitamin C with bioflavonoids (1,000 mg daily), and vitamin E (400 IU daily).

OTHER HELPFUL INFORMATION

Genital herpes can be especially harmful to a fetus. If you are pregnant, avoid contracting herpes because getting the disease poses a risk of transmitting it to your baby. If you get the disease early in pregnancy, your body has time to develop antibodies to the virus and so passes those antibodies along to your child. If you get the disease later in pregnancy, you won't have the antibodies, and so you will likely undergo a cesarean section to avoid transmitting the disease to your child.

READ MORE ABOUT IT

Ebel, Charles. *Managing Herpes: Living and Loving with HSV.* American Social Health Association, 2007.

ICON Health Publications. *The Official Patient's Sourcebook on Genital Herpes: A Revised and Updated Directory for the Internet Age.* ICON Health Publications, 2002.

Vynograd N et al. A comparative multi-centre study of the efficacy of propolis, acyclovir and placebo in the treatment of genital herpes (HSV). *Phytomedicine* 2000 Mar; 7(1):1–6.

GONORRHEA

Gonorrhea is the second most commonly reported sexually transmitted disease in the United States, with chlamydia holding the number one spot. More than 700,000 people get gonorrhea each year in the United States, but about 80 percent of women do not experience symptoms, which means they are unaware they have the disease and so do not seek treatment. When symptoms do occur, they may include a burning sensation when urinating, increased vaginal discharge, or bleeding between periods. If the rectum is infected, the most common symptoms are anal itching, soreness, bleeding, or painful bowel movements.

Gonorrhea is spread through contact with the vagina, penis, anus, or mouth, and it can also be spread from a mother to her infant during delivery. Although anyone who is sexually active can contract the disease, it is most often found in teenagers, young adults, and African Americans.

CAUSES AND RISK FACTORS
Gonorrhea is caused by the bacterium *Neisseria gonorrhoeae,* an organism that cannot exist outside the body for more than a few seconds. That means gonorrhea cannot be transmitted on toilet seats, towels, or other objects that have been touched by someone who has the disease. You place yourself in jeopardy for getting the disease if you have unprotected sex out-

side of a committed monogamous relationship and/or you have many sexual partners.

DIAGNOSIS
If you have symptoms of gonorrhea and/or you have any reason to suspect you may have contracted the disease, see a physician immediately. Diagnosis of gonorrhea requires health care professionals to take one or more samples for laboratory evaluation and, in most cases, to do a bimanual pelvic examination to determine if the fallopian tubes have been infected. In most cases, physicians use a speculum and swab to take a sample of cervical secretions, because the cervix is typically the first place the infection settles. A urine sample also can be used to test for gonorrhea in the cervix or urethra.

PREVENTION AND TREATMENT
Next to abstaining from sex, practicing safe sex is the best way to prevent getting gonorrhea. If you should get gonorrhea, antibiotics are used to treat and eliminate the infection. Antibiotics currently used to treat gonorrhea include ceftriaxone by injection followed by a one-week course of doxycycline orally. Alternatives to ceftriaxone include oral cefiximine, ciprofloxacin, or ofloxacin. If you are pregnant, you should not take ciprofloxacin, ofloxacin, or doxycycline (erythromycin can be substituted for doxycycline).

Both you and your sexual partner(s) should be tested and treated for gonorrhea, even if none of you has symptoms. You should avoid sexual contact until you and your partner(s) have been treated and the infection has been eliminated. Beware, however, that although you have been treated for gonorrhea, you can get reinfected if you have sexual contact with someone who has the disease.

OTHER HELPFUL INFORMATION
If you are pregnant and have untreated gonorrhea, you are at high risk for miscarriage or preterm delivery. You can also transmit the infection to your baby during vaginal delivery,

placing the infant at risk for blindness, joint infections, or a life-threatening blood infection. Infants born to mothers who have gonorrhea are treated with antibiotics and their eyes are treated with silver nitrate to prevent infection.

READ MORE ABOUT IT
ICON Health Publications. *Gonorrhea: A Medical Dictionary, Bibliography, and Annotated Research Guide to Internet References.* ICON Health Publications, 2004.

Newman LM et al. Update on the management of gonorrhea in adults in the United States. *Clin Infect Dis* 2007 Apr 1; 44 Suppl 3:S84–101.

INFERTILITY

Infertility is the diagnosis given when a couple is unsuccessful in their attempts to get pregnant after one year of unprotected sexual intercourse, or after six months of unprotected sex in women who are older than thirty-five. If the reason for the inability to conceive lies with the female, it is called female infertility. Female infertility factors contribute to about half of all infertility cases, and female infertility is the only reason in about one-third of all infertility cases. About 10 percent of American couples face the challenge of infertility.

CAUSES AND RISK FACTORS
Common causes of infertility in women include hormone dysfunction, which can halt ovulation or cause the eggs to be inadequate; pelvic inflammatory disease; fibroids; endometriosis; malformation of the fallopian tubes or uterus; anorexia nervosa; inflammation or other disorders affecting the cervix; an immunologic reaction that causes the woman's body to produce antibodies to the male's sperm; or certain medications (e.g., antibiotics can prevent embryo implantation; aspirin, ibuprofen, and antidepressants can suppress ovulation).

DIAGNOSIS
To determine the cause of infertility in women, an infertility specialist, either a reproductive endocrinologist or a sterologist, is usually consulted (see the section on reproductive

endocrinologists in "How to Find the Right Health Care Professional" in Part III). These individuals conduct comprehensive history and physical examinations and collect urine and blood samples. A basal body temperature should be done to determine if ovulation has occurred; blood tests are needed to determine hormone levels; tests to check for fallopian tube obstruction and cervical mucus receptibility to sperm are done; and sperm viability and compatibility are evaluated.

PREVENTION AND TREATMENT

Most cases of female infertility are beyond basic methods of prevention. However, you can definitely practice lifestyle habits that promote a healthy environment for conception; that is, don't smoke, minimize use of caffeine and alcohol, avoid exposure to environmental toxins, cease any recreational drug use, maintain a healthy weight, follow a nutritious diet, and manage stress in healthy ways.

Treatment depends on the cause of the infertility. Antibiotics may be necessary to eliminate pelvic inflammatory disease and cervical or uterine infections, for example, while uterine fibroids may be corrected by surgery. If your partner's semen analysis is normal but the evaluation of your cervical mucus test is not, your doctor may suggest estrogen therapy or artificial insemination. Ovulation can be induced or improved by taking clomiphene citrate, human menopausal gonadotropin, or other fertility drugs. For some women, an embryo transplant procedure may be needed (see "In Vitro Fertilization" in Part II).

SELF-HELP AND COMPLEMENTARY CARE

In addition to the lifestyle suggestions under "Prevention and Treatment," some complementary approaches may be helpful. Herbal remedies have been used for millennia to treat infertility, and today experts find that they seem to work best in women who have irregular menstrual cycles or hormone imbalances. To get the most from herbal remedies for infertility, you should consult a knowledgeable naturopath or herbalist who can recommend the right formula for you. This is critical because herbs, although natural, are potent and interact in negative ways with some medications, treatments, and supplements.

Herbal therapies for infertility often contain many ingredients that are available in pills, tablets, teas, or granules. Some of the more commonly used herbs to treat female infertility include black cohosh, chasteberry, dong quai, false unicorn root, licorice, red clover blossom, and wild yam.

OTHER HELPFUL INFORMATION

Preliminary evidence indicates that acupuncture, when combined with in vitro fertilization, may improve your chances of getting pregnant, according to a review conducted by the University of Maryland School of Medicine of seven studies that included more than 1,300 women. Acupuncture is also often combined with herbal remedies to treat unexplained infertility and some specific causes of infertility, such as polycystic ovarian syndrome. Exactly why acupuncture works for infertility problems is debatable, although acupuncturists claim that the therapy helps balance and regulate the body's blood flow and hormone levels, both of which can improve your chances of getting pregnant.

READ MORE ABOUT IT

Domar, Alice. *Conquering Infertility: Dr. Alice Domar's Mind/Body Guide to Enhancing Fertility and Coping with Infertility*. Penguin, 2004.

Lewis, Randine. *The Infertility Cure: The Ancient Chinese Wellness Program for Getting Pregnant and Having Healthy Babies*. Little, Brown, 2005.

Manheimer E et al. Effects of acupuncture on rates of pregnancy and live birth among women undergoing in vitro fertilisation: systematic review and meta-analysis. *BMJ* 2008 Mar 8; 336(7643): 545–49.

INFLAMMATION OF THE BREAST (MASTITIS)

Inflammation of the breast, or mastitis, is most often seen in breast-feeding women. Symptoms include pain in the affected breast, redness, tenderness, and swelling. Most women also experience general malaise, chills, and fever, which can soar quite high. If mastitis is treated promptly, it usually disappears within about forty-eight hours of starting treatment. If it is neglected, however, an abscess can develop, which may need to be drained.

At one time, moms with mastitis were told to stop breast-feeding to prevent infecting their baby. However, experts now recognize that breast-feeding can continue since the bacteria that caused the infection usually came from the baby's mouth. In addition, many women with mastitis say that breast-feeding relieves the pain by emptying the breast.

CAUSES AND RISK FACTORS

Mastitis is usually caused by the bacteria *Staphylococcus aureus,* but other organisms may be the culprits as well. The bacteria typically enter the breast through a crack in the nipple from the mouth of a suckling infant, although a love bite or other break in the nipple may be the source of the bacteria as well.

You increase your risk of getting mastitis if you:

• Use only one position to breast-feed

• Have a history of mastitis

- Have cracked or sore nipples

- Wear tight-fitting bras, which can restrict milk flow

DIAGNOSIS
A diagnosis of mastitis can be made by a physician based on your signs and symptoms. Contact your doctor as soon as you develop indications of mastitis so you can be treated to avoid development of an abscess.

PREVENTION AND TREATMENT
You can minimize your chances of getting mastitis if you practice these breast-feeding tips:

- Allow your infant to completely empty one breast before you switch him or her to the other breast.

- Alternate the breast you offer first at each feeding.

- Change your feeding position at each session.

- Make sure your infant latches on properly at each feeding.

- Do not let your baby use your breast as a pacifier.

Conventional medical treatment of mastitis is with oral antibiotics for ten to fourteen days and warm compresses. Although you will probably feel better twenty-four to forty-eight hours after starting the antibiotics, you should take the entire course of medication to prevent recurrence.

SELF-HELP AND COMPLEMENTARY CARE
Women have been using natural remedies for mastitis for millennia. Although their methods have not been proven scientifically, they have the endorsement of countless numbers of women. One popular remedy is to place raw cabbage leaves on the affected breast. You can slip a leaf into your bra and

replace it every few hours. This cure is reportedly especially effective when a duct just becomes clogged and before infection sets in. If you feel odd doing this, just remember that no one needs to know!

A less exotic remedy is echinacea root tincture, one full dropper six times daily until the fever has passed, and then take two or three times daily until all the symptoms have been eliminated. Yet another approach is a comfrey and calendula poultice, which can help draw out the infection. To make the poultice, put equal amounts of comfrey leaves and calendula flowers into a blender with a small amount of water and a tablespoon of flour. Process until it has a gelatinlike form. Spread some of the poultice onto a cotton cloth, heat it in the oven or microwave until comfortably warm, and place it on the affected breast. Apply the poultice at least four times daily until the symptoms clear.

READ MORE ABOUT IT

Betzold CM. An update on the recognition and management of lactational breast inflammation. *J Midwifery Womens Health* 2007 Nov–Dec; 52(6): 595–605.

MISCARRIAGE

A miscarriage is the involuntary loss of a pregnancy without obvious reason before the twentieth week of pregnancy. The American College of Obstetricians and Gynecologists estimates that 15 percent of known pregnancies end in miscarriage, but the actual number is likely much higher because many miscarriages occur early in pregnancy even before a woman knows she is pregnant.

In fact, most miscarriages occur before the twelfth week of pregnancy. Signs and symptoms of a miscarriage are vaginal spotting or bleeding, fluid or tissue passing from the vagina, and pain or cramping in the abdomen or lower back. Spotting or bleeding early in pregnancy is common, and most women who bleed during their first trimester have successful pregnancies. Therefore bleeding is not an automatic indication that a miscarriage is occurring.

CAUSES AND RISK FACTORS

Most miscarriages occur because the fetus is not developing normally. This is usually related to problems with the infant's genes or chromosomes that arose as the embryo divided and grew, and not genetic problems inherited from the parents. In a small percentage of cases, a mother's health problems—thyroid disease, blood-clotting problems, infections, problems with the uterus or cervix, uncontrolled diabetes—may result in miscarriage. Activities that do not prompt a miscarriage—

these are old wives' tales—include having sex, exercising, lifting heavy objects, and nausea and vomiting in early pregnancy. A fall or other injury in most cases will not cause a miscarriage unless the injury is life-threatening to the woman.

Risk factors for miscarriage include the following:

- **Age.** Women older than thirty-five have a greater risk of miscarriage than do younger women, as do women whose partners are age forty or older.

- **Previous miscarriages.** A history of two or more miscarriages increases your risk for another.

- **Chronic illness.** Women who have a chronic condition such as diabetes, thyroid disease, or lupus have a higher risk of miscarriage.

- **Alcohol, smoking, and drugs.** Use of alcohol, tobacco, and/or illicit drugs increases the risk of miscarriage.

- **Caffeine.** The impact of caffeine on miscarriage is not known for certain. Many doctors recommend that pregnant women avoid caffeine during their first trimester and limit themselves to 300 mg daily during the remainder of the pregnancy.

- **Cervical or uterine problems.** A weak or unusually short cervix and certain uterine abnormalities may increase the risk of miscarriage.

DIAGNOSIS

If you are pregnant and experiencing signs or symptoms of miscarriage—vaginal bleeding, pain or cramping in your lower back or abdomen—contact your doctor immediately. You may need to undergo a pelvic exam to see if your cervix is dilating. Your doctor may do an ultrasound to check for a fetal heartbeat and determine if the embryo is developing normally. Blood and urine tests also may be ordered.

Often there is bleeding but the cervix has not begun to dilate. This is called a threatened miscarriage, and most of these pregnancies proceed to term without problems. In such cases, many doctors recommend resting until the bleeding or pain disappears, and to avoid exercise, sex, and traveling. If, however, you are experiencing contractions and your cervix is dilating, the miscarriage is inevitable.

PREVENTION AND TREATMENT
In most cases, there is nothing you can do to prevent a miscarriage. Naturally, you should avoid the known risk factors, such as alcohol and smoking, and you should get regular prenatal care. Some research indicates that taking aspirin or another type of blood thinner to prevent blood clots may improve your chances of a successful pregnancy if you have had unexplained miscarriages in the past. You can discuss this possibility with your physician.

When a miscarriage is inevitable, or after a miscarriage occurs, there are various treatment options you can consider.

- **Expectant management.** If you have an ultrasound and it shows a miscarriage before you have experienced any signs or symptoms, you may choose to let the miscarriage happen naturally. This natural progression typically occurs within a few weeks of discovering that the embryo has died.

- **Medical approach.** If the miscarriage is inevitable and you want to accelerate the process, your doctor can give you a medication that will cause your body to eliminate the pregnancy tissue and placenta. The medication can be taken either orally or vaginally, and most doctors recommend the latter because it is both more effective and associated with milder side effects. Reactions to the medication may include nausea, vomiting, cramping, and diarrhea. The exact timing of the miscarriage after taking the medication varies.

- **Surgical approach.** If your cervix is dilated and you are bleeding, are in pain, or have had a miscarriage but some tissue remains behind, you may need a minor surgical procedure called a dilatation and curettage (D&C; see "Dilatation and Curettage" in Part II). Complications are rare but may include damage to the cervix or uterine wall.

SELF-HELP AND COMPLEMENTARY CARE

When a miscarriage occurs, emotional support is critical. You will likely experience a wide range of emotions, from anger to despair to depression. This is a time to seek emotional support from those you love and who love you, and perhaps to turn to professionals as well—a religious or spiritual leader, a grief counselor, a loss support group, or a psychologist. Allow yourself time to grieve the loss of your child.

OTHER HELPFUL INFORMATION

Many women wonder how long after a miscarriage they should wait until they get pregnant again. It's possible to become pregnant during the menstrual cycle that immediately follows a miscarriage. You and your partner should be sure, however, that you are both emotionally and physically ready for another pregnancy. Your doctor may recommend that you wait for more than one menstrual cycle. This is also a question you can discuss with your loved ones and spiritual advisor if you have one.

READ MORE ABOUT IT

Beer, Alan E., MD. *Is Your Body Baby-Friendly? Unexplained Infertility, Miscarriage, and IVF Failure—Explained and Treated.* AJR, 2006.

Rousselot, Susan. *Avoiding Miscarriage: Everything You Need to Know to Feel More Confident in Pregnancy.* Sea Change Press, 2006.

OVARIAN CYSTS

An ovarian cyst is a fluid-filled sac that develops on the ovaries. These growths can develop at any age, occur alone or in clusters, and can affect one or both ovaries. They are relatively common, and most of them cause little or no discomfort and are harmless. In fact, the majority of ovarian cysts disappear without treatment within a few months of their appearance.

Some women develop less common types of ovarian cysts that often do not produce symptoms, but your doctor may discover them during a pelvic examination. Ovarian cysts that develop after menopause may be cancerous, and so it is important to keep having regular pelvic examinations.

CAUSES AND RISK FACTORS
Several different types of cysts can form on the ovaries, and each one develops for a different reason.

- **Follicular cysts,** which form during the normal menstrual cycle. A follicle is the fluid-filled sac that contains en egg, and the follicle is supposed to burst and release the egg. However, if it fails to open and grows larger than normal, it can develop into a cyst, which usually disappears within one to three months.

- **Corpus luteum cysts**, which also form during the normal menstrual cycle. In this case, the sac fails to dissolve after releasing the egg, and fluid accumulates inside the sac. This type of cyst may disappear after several weeks or continue to grow and cause pain and bleeding.

- **Endometriomas** develop in women who have endometriosis. These can be painful during menstruation and sexual intercourse.

- **Cystadenomas** occur on the outer surface of the ovary. They can grow to be large (up to 12 inches in diameter) and painful.

- **Dermoid cysts** are both uncommon and unusual in that they contain very diverse tissues, including hair, bone, thyroid, and teeth. They can range in size from 1 cm (less than 0.5 inch) up to 45 cm (about 17 inches) in diameter. The larger the cyst, the more likely it is to cause the ovary to twist and thus jeopardize its blood supply. This is a situation that requires immediate medical attention.

- **Polycystic ovaries** occur when the eggs mature with the sacs each month but the sacs don't release them, and so they accumulate and cysts form. See "Polycystic Ovary Syndrome."

DIAGNOSIS
Because ovarian cysts often do not cause symptoms, they are usually discovered during a pelvic exam. If your doctor does feel a swelling on your ovary, he or she may recommend having an ultrasound, which can reveal the shape, location, and size of the cyst, and whether it is solid, filled with fluid, or mixed. Your doctor may also order blood tests to check your hormone levels. If you are older than thirty-five and have a cyst that is partially solid, your doctor may order another blood test to detect levels of CA-125, a protein that is present in elevated

levels if a woman has endometrial cancer or endometriosis (see "Endometrial Cancer" and "Endometriosis").

PREVENTION AND TREATMENT
Although ovarian cysts cannot be prevented, the good news is that most of them are not cancerous, they eventually disappear on their own, and they don't cause significant symptoms. If treatment is necessary, however, there are several alternatives.

If you are of childbearing age, have no symptoms, and have a fluid-filled cyst, your doctor may recommend getting reexamined in one to three months to see if the cyst has changed in size. In many cases the cyst gradually shrinks and disappears. If, however, after several menstrual cycles the cyst remains unchanged, has grown, causes pain, or appears unusual on ultrasound, your doctor may want to remove it. Surgery is often recommended as well for postmenopausal women with an ovarian cyst.

Two types of surgery can be done. If the cyst is small and looks benign on the ultrasound, a laparoscopy, which requires a tiny incision, can be done. A recent study shows, however, that large, benign ovarian cysts can be successfully removed by laparoscopy as well. If the cyst is large and may be cancerous, the doctor may perform a laparotomy, which involves a larger incision. If you have recurring cysts, your doctor may recommend taking birth control pills to reduce your chances of forming new cysts.

SELF-HELP AND COMPLEMENTARY CARE
If you are experiencing pain associated with an ovarian cyst, an herbal remedy to relieve discomfort is chamomile and ginger root tea: steep 1 teaspoon of each dried herb in 8 ounces of hot water for five to ten minutes and drink two to four cups daily. Some naturopaths also recommend taking chasteberry tincture (50 to 60 drops daily) to help shrink small cysts.

Although there are no scientific studies to back up the claims made by homeopaths, there are anecdotal reports that

combination homeopathic remedies that contain apis, colo-
cynthis, lachesis, and lodum may provide relief from symptoms. Consult a knowledgeable homeopath for guidance on
the right combination for you.

READ MORE ABOUT IT

Eltabbakh GH et al. Laparoscopic surgery for large benign
ovarian cysts. *Gynecol Oncol* 2008 Jan; 108(1): 72–76.

Stany MP, Hamilton CA. Benign disorders of the ovary.
Obstet Gynecol Clin North Am 2008 Jun; 35(2): 271–84.

PAINFUL MENSTRUATION (MENORRHAGIA)

Painful menstruation, also known as menorrhagia or hypermenorrhea, is abnormally heavy bleeding during regular menstrual periods. While the typical menstrual blood loss is 4 to 12 teaspoons (20 to 60 grams) per cycle, menorrhagia is defined as losing 80 ml or more. Women who have menorrhagia typically have menstrual periods that last longer than seven days, need to change tampons or sanitary pads every hour for several consecutive hours, pass large blood clots, and experience constant pain in the lower abdomen during their period. Some complain of fatigue, shortness of breath, and tiredness, which are all symptoms of anemia.

CAUSES AND RISK FACTORS

All women of reproductive age are at risk of menorrhagia, but the risk is greater among women as they approach menopause, women who have a hereditary bleeding disorder, and young women who have just begun menstruation.

Menorrhagia can be caused by a long list of factors, including hormone imbalance, uterine fibroids, adenomyosis, use of an IUD, certain medications (e.g., anticoagulants, some anti-inflammatories), pelvic inflammatory disease, endometriosis, thyroid problems, and polyps.

DIAGNOSIS

The only way to make an accurate diagnosis of menorrhagia is to rule out other menstrual disorders (e.g., those named under "Causes and Risk Factors"), medical conditions, or medications that could be causing or aggravating your symptoms. To do that, your doctor will conduct or order one or more of the following:

- Blood tests to look for blood-clotting problems or thyroid disorders

- Pap test to detect inflammation, infections, or cancerous changes

- Ultrasound scan of the uterus, pelvis, and ovaries to look for growths or other abnormalities

- Endometrial biopsy to check uterine health

- Hysteroscopy to look inside the uterus

- Sonohysterogram to look at the lining of the uterus

- Dilation and curettage to collect tissue samples from the uterus

PREVENTION AND TREATMENT

Although menorrhagia is not preventable, it is treatable. Given the many possible causes for the condition, there are a varied number of treatments available. Nonsteroidal anti-inflammatory drugs (NSAIDs) are usually recommended to relieve painful menstrual cramps, while oral contraceptives may be prescribed to help regulate ovulation and reduce excessive bleeding. Use of progesterone alone also may correct hormonal imbalances and reduce cramping. If excessive bleeding has left you with anemia, your doctor may prescribe iron supplements (but have your iron levels checked before beginning supplementation).

If these methods have not provided relief, your doctor may recommend one of the following surgical procedures:

- **Dilatation and curettage (D&C).** Scraping of tissue from the uterine lining, which reduces menstrual bleeding. Although this procedure is often successful for a time, it may need to be repeated in subsequent years.

- **Endometrial ablation.** Use of ultrasound to eliminate the uterine lining (endometrium), which may result in normal, limited, or no menstrual flow.

- **Endometrial resection.** Like endometrial ablation, this removes the lining of the uterus.

- **Hysterectomy.** Surgical removal of the uterus and cervix. Removal of the ovaries and uterus (oophorohysterectomy) may cause premature menopause in younger women. A laparoscopic hysterectomy is available and can significantly reduce recovery time.

- **Operative hysteroscopy.** Used to remove polyps.

SELF-HELP AND COMPLEMENTARY CARE
Because heavy menstrual flow increases your risk for iron-deficiency anemia, increase your dietary iron intake rather than resort to iron supplements (unless deemed necessary by your doctor). Symptoms of iron-deficiency anemia include paleness, weakness, and fatigue. Foods rich in iron include bran flakes, chickpeas, eggs, lentils, liver, oatmeal, prunes, sea vegetables, and tofu. Be sure to eat foods rich in vitamin C along with these foods, as vitamin C enhances iron absorption.

OTHER HELPFUL INFORMATION
Avoid taking aspirin, as it interferes with blood clotting. To help both you and your doctor determine how much blood

you lose during each period, record the number of pads and tampons you use.

READ MORE ABOUT IT

ICON Health Publications. *Menorrhagia: A Medical Dictionary, Bibliography, and Annotated Research Guide to Internet References.* ICON Health Publications, 2004.

Erian J et al. Efficacy of laparoscopic subtotal hysterectomy in the management of menorrhagia: 400 consecutive cases. *BJOG* 2008 May; 115(6): 742–48.

PAINFUL SEXUAL INTERCOURSE (DYSPAREUNIA)

Painful sexual intercourse, or dyspareunia, is a condition in which women experience persistent or recurring pain just before, during, or after sexual intercourse. Dyspareunia can be caused by a wide variety of factors, both physical and emotional, and it is a phenomenon shared by many women. Yet women tend to suffer in silence, and most do not seek medical help because they are embarrassed to talk to their health care providers about sex or they've been told that it's "all in their head."

Perhaps the most important things to know about dyspareunia is that *it is real; it is not just in your head;* and in nearly every case *treatment can eliminate or reduce symptoms.* Sex should be pleasurable, not painful, and a knowledgeable and understanding health professional can help you address this problem so you can better enjoy sexual activity.

CAUSES AND RISK FACTORS
Some of the more common causes of dyspareunia include the following:

- Insufficient lubrication/vaginal dryness

- Allergic reaction to latex and/or spermicide

- Bacterial or yeast infection, including chlamydia, vaginitis, and vaginosis

- Endometriosis

- Retroverted or tipped uterus

- Low estrogen levels (common during menopause and postmenopause)

- Pelvic inflammatory disease

- Ovarian cysts or fibroids

- Vulvodynia

- Drugs to treat high blood pressure, depression, and allergies, among others, can cause vaginal dryness and/or reduce sex drive

- Muscle spasms around the vagina (see "Painful Vaginal Spasms")

Emotional or psychological issues (e.g., history of sexual abuse or rape, fear of sex, guilty feelings about sex) also may cause or be a risk factor for dyspareunia for some women.

DIAGNOSIS

To determine the cause of your pain, your doctor will likely ask you questions about your symptoms, sexual history, and any other concerns or problems you may have with sex. Telling your doctor exactly when you experience the pain—before entry, with entry, or once the penis is in the vagina—can provide him or her with important clues about the cause. For most women, pain occurs with vaginal entry. Your doctor will likely do a genital or an internal pelvic exam, and based on those findings, you may be asked to undergo testing for bacterial or yeast infection, urinalysis, or allergy testing.

PREVENTION AND TREATMENT
Prevention and treatment will depend on your diagnosis. You can get details by referring to the appropriate entries (e.g., "Endometriosis," "Pelvic Inflammatory Disease," "Vaginitis").

SELF-HELP AND COMPLEMENTARY CARE
Self-help and complementary care may be recommended, depending on your diagnosis. See the appropriate individual entries and the suggestions for each one.

OTHER HELPFUL INFORMATION
Research shows that up to 60 percent of women experience dyspareunia, yet many women who have persistent symptoms do not seek medical or psychological help. The embarrassment, guilt, or shame that women feel about this condition often has a significant impact on their relationship with their sex partner. Thus dyspareunia is a condition that affects both people in a sexual relationship and, if unresolved, may place a great deal of stress on the partnership. For some women, talking with a sex therapist, couples counselor, marriage counselor, or other mental health professional, along with their partner, provides good results. See the Appendix for mental health resources.

READ MORE ABOUT IT
Frank JE et al. Diagnosis and treatment of female sexual dysfunction. *Am Fam Physician* 2008 Mar 1; 77(5): 635–42.

Glatt AE et al. The prevalence of dyspareunia. *Obstet Gynecol* 1990 Mar; 75(3 Pt 1): 433–36.

PM Medical Health News. *21st Century Complete Medical Guide to Female Sexual Dysfunction, Dyspareunia, Authoritative Government Documents, Clinical References, and Practical Information for Patients and Physicians.* Progressive Management, 2004.

PAINFUL VAGINAL SPASMS (VAGINISMUS)

Vaginismus is a condition in which the vagina involuntarily tightens during attempted sexual intercourse. Women who have this condition often are not even aware that this involuntary response by the pelvic floor muscles is the reason for the problems they are having during sexual intercourse. For some women, vaginismus begins as a burning or stinging pain during intercourse. For others, penetration is very difficult or impossible because the vagina is so "closed" that the man is unable to insert his penis.

It is difficult to know how many women suffer with vaginismus. Generally, experts believe that 2 of every 1,000 women have the condition, although numbers understandably are much greater depending on the population surveyed. At the Sexual Dysfunction Clinic at Loyola University in Chicago, for example, the incidence rate of vaginismus among its clients was given as 7 percent, while a survey revealed that 16 percent of women who consulted with one birth control clinic were suffering from vaginismus.

CAUSES AND RISK FACTORS

Possible causes of vaginismus include both physical and psychological factors. Women who have cystitis, a vaginal infection, or endometriosis, for example, may experience vaginismus. Psychological causes may include fear of pain, fear of painful sex, fear of pregnancy, strict religious upbringing, early childhood trauma, experiences with painful penetration (from sex, use of tampons, pelvic examination), and rape.

DIAGNOSIS
The official criterion for the diagnosis of vaginismus is the involuntary, recurring, or persistent spasm of the muscles in the outer third of the vagina. Diagnosing sexual disorders such as vaginismus can be difficult because many women are not comfortable discussing their sexual relations with their physicians. A pelvic examination can usually confirm the diagnosis, because women with the disorder will have an involuntary spasm during the exam. It is also important for the doctor to review a woman's medical history and do a complete physical examination to rule out other possible causes for the pain.

PREVENTION AND TREATMENT
Because vaginismus often has a psychological component, even if the cause is physical, treatment should include counseling (couples therapy, group therapy, individual counseling), education, and behavioral exercises, such as Kegel exercises. Health care practitioners may also recommend vaginal dilation exercises, which use plastic dilators to help women gradually relax and allow penetration. These exercises should be done under the guidance of a sex therapist or other qualified health care professional. Educational materials should be shared and explained to both the woman and her partner. This combination of approaches can be very successful.

SELF-HELP AND COMPLEMENTARY CARE
Some women have had success using hypnotherapy to overcome vaginismus. This approach is not for everyone, and a qualified therapist can determine if it is right. Generally, the woman and her hypnotherapist work to define the goals of therapy and the suggestions that will be made during hypnosis before the actual hypnosis occurs. During hypnosis, the issues that are behind the vaginismus may be explored or the hypnotherapist may work to eliminate the fears that may be

causing the disorder. If you want to work with a hypnothera-pist, make sure you find one who is familiar with sexual disor-ders and who has credentials. Although only one state licenses hypnotherapists (California), you should look for a hypno-therapist who has been certified by the National Guild of Hypnotists or another recognized institution or organization.

READ MORE ABOUT IT

Kleinplatz PJ. Sex therapy for vaginismus: a review, critique, and humanistic alternative. *J Humanistic Psychol* 1998; 38(2): 51–82.

Reissing ED et al. Vaginal spasm, pain, and behavior: an empirical investigation of the diagnosis of vaginismus. *Arch Sex Behav* 2004 Feb; 33(1): 5–17.

Valins, Linda. *When a Woman's Body Says No to Sex: Under-standing and Overcoming Vaginismus.* Penguin Books, 1992.

PELVIC INFLAMMATORY DISEASE (PID)

Pelvic inflammatory disease (PID) is a general term for a common infection of the uterus, fallopian tubes, and other reproductive organs. This potentially serious disease can lead to infertility, ectopic pregnancy, abscesses, and chronic pelvic pain. More than 1 million women experience an episode of PID each year, and more than 100,000 women become infertile as a result of having the disease.

CAUSES AND RISK FACTORS
Pelvic inflammatory disease can develop when bacteria travel up from the vagina or cervix into the rest of the reproductive organs. Various organisms can cause this condition, but two common sexually transmitted diseases—chlamydia and gonorrhea—are associated with many cases of PID.

You are more likely to get PID if you have a history of the disease, if you have many sexual partners, and if you are younger than twenty-five, partly because the cervix of young women is not fully matured, which increases its susceptibility to STDs that are associated with PID. Douching also increases your risk because it can create an unhealthy environment in the vagina and force bacteria past the vagina into other reproductive organs.

DIAGNOSIS
Many women and their health care providers don't recognize cases of PID because the symptoms are often mild and

nonspecific. This fact, as well as the lack of precise tests for PID, make diagnosis difficult. Diagnosis is usually based on clinical findings, such as evidence of chlamydial infection or abnormal vaginal discharge. A pelvic ultrasound can help diagnose PID, because it can detect abscesses and enlarged fallopian tubes. Some women require a laparoscopy to confirm the diagnosis.

PREVENTION AND TREATMENT

You can protect yourself from getting PID by taking steps to prevent STDs. The best way to avoid getting STDs is to abstain from sexual intercourse or to be in a long-term mutually monogamous relationship with a partner who is not infected. If you should contract an STD, get immediate treatment to ward off PID. Consistent and correct use of latex male condoms can also reduce your risk of getting STDs.

Antibiotics are necessary to eliminate PID, and doctors typically prescribe more than one because more than one organism is usually involved. Therefore, broad-spectrum oral antibiotics are usually started immediately after you get your diagnosis and continued for about two weeks. If you have a severe case, if you are pregnant, or if you have an abscess in your fallopian tubes or ovary, your doctor may admit you to the hospital for treatment. If you are treated at home, however, you should get plenty of bed rest for several days to help prevent further inflammation of the uterus and fallopian tubes. Although antibiotics can eliminate the infection, they cannot reverse any damage that the bacteria already caused to the reproductive organs.

SELF-HELP AND COMPLEMENTARY CARE

To help reduce inflammation naturally, some naturopaths suggest taking bromelain (500 mg three times per day between meals), curcumin (500 mg three times daily), or flaxseed oil (1,500 mg two or three times daily). For best results, take bromelain and curcumin together to enhance anti-inflammatory effects.

OTHER HELPFUL INFORMATION

Left untreated, PID can cause permanent damage to your reproductive organs. For example, the bacteria can scar your fallopian tubes, making it difficult or impossible for eggs to be transported into the uterus. If the scar tissue completely blocks the fallopian tubes, you can become infertile, although infertility can also occur even if the tubes are only partially blocked. About 10 percent of women who have PID become infertile (see "Infertility").

If a fertilized egg becomes stuck in a partially blocked or damaged fallopian tube, the egg can grow in the tube, resulting in an ectopic pregnancy. As the embryo develops, an ectopic pregnancy can rupture the fallopian tube, causing severe pain, bleeding, and even death (see "Ectopic Pregnancy").

READ MORE ABOUT IT

Evans DT et al. A retrospective audit of the management and complications of pelvic inflammatory disease. *Int J STD AIDS* 2008 Feb; 19(2): 123–24.

O'Donnell, Judith A. *Pelvic Inflammatory Disease*. Chelsea House Publications, 2006.

Pelvic Organ Prolapse. *See* "Prolapsed Bladder (Cystocele)"

POLYCYSTIC OVARY SYNDROME (PCOS)

Polycystic ovary syndrome (PCOS) is a condition in which women have many small cysts (fluid-filled sacs) in their ovaries. This disorder is accompanied by a long list of symptoms, including irregular menstrual periods, high cholesterol, high blood pressure, acne, weight gain, insulin resistance, pelvic pain, anxiety, sleep apnea, thinning hair, and hair growth on the face, chest, stomach, and back. Ten percent of women of child-bearing age have polycystic ovary syndrome, a source of distress for many of them because this condition is the number one cause of female infertility.

In polycystic ovary syndrome, the body produces an abnormally high amount of male hormones, called androgens, and ovulation (the release of eggs by the ovaries) occurs irregularly or not at all. When ovulation is irregular, so is the menstrual cycle.

CAUSES AND RISK FACTORS
Experts do not know what causes polycystic ovary syndrome, but research indicates that women with this condition have an excessive amount of insulin, and the abnormally high level may cause androgen production to increase. Some studies also suggest that genetics play a role.

DIAGNOSIS

Diagnosing polycystic ovary syndrome is done mainly by process of elimination, since there are no definitive tests for the condition. Basically your doctor will consider all your signs and symptoms, conduct a physical examination, including a pelvic examination, and may include other tests:

- Blood tests may be done to measure hormone levels. Levels of male hormones (e.g., testosterone, DHEA) tend to be high in PCOS, as does the ratio of luteinizing hormone and follicle-stimulating hormone.

- Blood tests may also be ordered to determine cholesterol, triglyceride, and fasting glucose levels, especially since insulin resistance is one sign of the disease.

- A pelvic ultrasound can reveal the condition of the ovaries and the thickness of the uterine lining.

PREVENTION AND TREATMENT

Prevention and treatment of PCOS typically involves addressing individual symptoms, protecting heart health, and preventing diabetes. For example, more than 50 percent of women with PCOS will develop diabetes or prediabetes before age forty, approximately 70 percent have excess hair growth, 40 to 70 percent are obese, and most have high cholesterol and triglyceride levels. Women with PCOS are also four to seven times more likely to experience a heart attack than their peers who do not have PCOS. The risk of endometrial cancer is also greater among women who have PCOS.

Research shows that insulin-lowering medications (e.g., metformin, rosiglitazone, pioglitazone) are effective in women who have PCOS because they reduce blood pressure, triglyceride levels, excess hair growth, and obesity, while also helping to reestablish a normal ovulation schedule. Although these antidiabetes drugs lower high blood sugar levels in diabetics, they only lower insulin levels when nondiabetics take them. Some physicians prescribe oral contraceptives to help reduce male hormone production.

A recent development is ovarian drilling, a surgical procedure done during laparoscopy in which physicians use a laser or special needle to puncture the ovary four to ten times. This procedure significantly reduces male hormone levels within a few days. (See "Pelvic Laparoscopy" in Part II.)

SELF-HELP AND COMPLEMENTARY CARE

A nutritional supplement program followed for at least three months may make a significant difference in PCOS. Begin with a good multivitamin/mineral tablet, one that contains 100 percent or more of the Daily Value (DV) for major nutrients, including all vitamins and eight minerals (calcium, chromium, copper, magnesium, manganese, potassium, selenium, and zinc). Add to this the following supplements, keeping in mind that you should consider any amounts you are already taking in your multi-supplement: 200 mcg chromium, 30 mg zinc, 300 mg magnesium, 50 mg each of the B vitamins, and 30 mg coenzyme Q_{10} (coQ_{10}). The B vitamins can help control weight, while B_3 in particular helps keep blood sugar levels in balance. Magnesium helps with insulin resistance, while coQ_{10} is important for energy production and carbohydrate metabolism. It also helps to control blood sugar levels.

OTHER HELPFUL INFORMATION

If you have PCOS and you want to become pregnant, you may need fertility medication. If you become pregnant, having PCOS places you at increased risk of gestational diabetes and pregnancy-induced high blood pressure. Discuss these and other possible complications with your health care provider.

READ MORE ABOUT IT

Elsheikh, M., and Caroline Murphy. *Polycystic Ovary Syndrome*. Oxford University Press, 2008.

Futterweit, W. *A Patient's Guide to PCOS: Understanding and Reversing Polycystic Ovary Syndrome.* Holt, 2006.

Johnson A et al. Current diagnosis and treatment of polycystic ovary syndrome. *S D Med* 2008 Apr; 61(4): 129, 131, 133.

PREECLAMPSIA

Preeclampsia, also known as toxemia, is a serious condition that occurs only during pregnancy and the postpartum period. This rapidly progressive condition affects at least 5 to 8 percent of all pregnant women. Typically it develops around week 20 of pregnancy, but it can occur earlier.

Signs and symptoms include elevated blood pressure (140/90 or higher), protein in the urine, sudden weight gain, headaches, changes in vision, and swelling of the hands, feet, and/or face. The earlier preeclampsia occurs in pregnancy, the greater the risks for the mother and her infant. Complications of preeclampsia include:

- **Interrupted blood flow to the placenta.** Preeclampsia can severely limit the amount of blood that flows through the placenta to the fetus. A fetus that does not get adequate nutrients or oxygen may experience slow growth, be born before term, have a low birth weight, or be stillborn.

- **HELLP syndrome.** This syndrome includes hemolysis (red blood cell destruction), elevated liver enzymes, and low platelet count, and is characterized by nausea, vomiting, headache, and upper right abdominal pain.

- **Placental abruption.** Preeclampsia increases the chance that the placenta will separate from the uterine wall (placental abruption) before delivery. This can cause heavy bleeding and threaten the life of both mother and child.

- **Eclampsia.** If preeclampsia is not controlled, eclampsia can develop. Symptoms include severe headache, vision problems, decreased alertness, and other changes in mental status. Eclampsia can permanently damage a mother's vital organs. If eclampsia is not treated, the condition can cause coma, brain damage, and death for both mother and infant.

CAUSES AND RISK FACTORS

The cause of this condition is not known. Experts have proposed several theories: some say preeclampsia is caused by an immune system dysfunction or there is a problem with blood clotting; others suggest genetics play a role or that abnormalities in the placenta are the key. Researchers do know that something causes the blood vessels to leak into the tissues, which then causes swelling in various places throughout the body. When the blood vessels leak into the kidneys, protein spills into the urine; when they leak into the liver, it can cause severe pain under the right side of the rib cage. When swelling occurs in the brain, seizures can occur. This condition is called eclampsia.

Preeclampsia occurs most often during first pregnancies, in women who are pregnant with twins or triplets, in teenagers or older women, and in women who have a history of preeclampsia. Between 10 and 15 percent of women get preeclampsia during their first pregnancy. Preeclampsia also appears to run in families.

DIAGNOSIS

A diagnosis of preeclampsia is given when a pregnant woman reaches at least twenty weeks' gestation and has high blood pressure (140/90 or greater) and protein in her urine. Because the liver and kidneys can be affected, doctors often monitor their function. To ensure the baby's health, doctors often use ultrasound to monitor growth and a nonstress test or biophysical profile to keep an eye on nourishment and oxygen intake.

PREVENTION AND TREATMENT
Since the cause of preeclampsia is not known, there is no way to prevent it except to not get pregnant. If you develop preeclampsia or eclampsia, the only real cure is to give birth. A mild case of preeclampsia (a small amount of protein in the urine and/or blood pressure greater than 140/90 that develops after twenty weeks of gestation in a woman with no history of hypertension) is usually treated with a watch-and-wait approach along with lots of rest and medication (if needed) if the baby is preterm. If the baby is close to term, the doctor may induce labor.

Women who have severe preeclampsia (lung problems, fetal distress, abdominal pain, vision problems) may need to have their child delivered immediately, regardless of the baby's age. In some cases, doctors may inject magnesium to prevent seizures or give hydralazine or another antihypertensive drug to manage severe high blood pressure.

SELF-HELP AND COMPLEMENTARY CARE
Think multiples! Taking multivitamins during pregnancy, especially those containing folic acid, can reduce the risk of preeclampsia. Both before and during pregnancy, women should get 800 mcg of folic acid daily. Experts already know that folic acid helps prevent birth defects, and you can add prevention of preeclampsia to the list as well. A 2008 University of Ottawa study of nearly 3,000 pregnant women found that those who took multivitamins containing folic acid during their second trimester had a reduced risk of developing preeclampsia.

Watching your weight is also recommended. In a 2006 study, women who took multivitamins and maintained a healthy weight before conception reduced their risk of developing preeclampsia during pregnancy by more than 70 percent when compared with women of a healthy weight who did not take vitamins or with women who took vitamins but who were overweight before getting pregnant.

OTHER HELPFUL INFORMATION

Although the research is preliminary, it appears that a vitamin D deficiency may put pregnant women at greater risk for preeclampsia. Since vitamin D is also essential for bone health, and because children born from mothers deficient in vitamin D have a higher risk of type 1 diabetes and bone mineral diseases, it is recommended that you get sufficient vitamin D (400–600 IU daily), especially before and during pregnancy.

READ MORE ABOUT IT

Bodnar LM et al. Maternal vitamin D deficiency increases the risk of preeclampsia. *J Clin Endocrinol Metab* 2007 Sep; 92(9): 3517–22.

PM Medical Health News. *21st Century Complete Medical Guide to Preeclampsia, Eclampsia, Toxemia of Pregnancy, Hypertension and Pregnancy, Authoritative Government Documents, Clinical Data and Practical Information for Patients and Physicians.* Progressive Management, 2004.

Wen SW et al. Folic acid supplementation in early second trimester and the risk of preeclampsia. *Am J Obstet Gynecol* 2008 Jan; 198(1): 45.e1–7.

PREGNANCY

Pregnancy is a condition in which a woman is carrying a fertilized egg, embryo, or fetus. That's a rather unsentimental definition for what is often a time of great joy and anticipation for many women and their partners. A full-term pregnancy continues for thirty-nine or forty weeks, which is divided into three 3-month periods called trimesters.

Pregnancy is characterized by a great number of physical and emotional changes that begin soon after conception. The earliest signs and symptoms of pregnancy are usually a skipped period, swollen and tender breasts, nausea, sleepiness and fatigue, increased vaginal discharge, slight cramping just above the pubis, and urinary frequency. Some women experience little beyond missed periods for the first few months; others struggle with morning sickness and fatigue every day.

All of these signs and symptoms are related to the hormonal changes that occur in a woman's body during pregnancy. Within five to seven days of conception, substances called chorionic gonadotropins appear in the blood and urine. These are the substances pregnancy tests are designed to detect. Estrogen and progesterone levels rise gradually. By week three or four, ultrasound can detect a fetus, and by week eleven, ultrasound can distinguish the mother's heartbeat from that of her fetus.

By the second trimester, the uterus has undergone tremendous changes in shape, size, and consistency. Pigment changes occur, especially darkening of the skin around the nipples and sometimes on the face. Stretch marks develop—as the skin over the growing abdomen is stretched, pink stretch marks are left behind. Varicose veins may develop in the legs. The 30 to 50 percent increase in blood volume that occurs during pregnancy causes the mother's heart to beat faster, and palpitations are common. Swollen ankles, feet, hands, and wrists are common.

By the third trimester, the considerably larger uterus and abdomen cause many women increasing discomfort. As the enlarged uterus pushes on other organs, many women experience shortness of breath, indigestion, constipation, urinary frequency, and pain associated with edema and varicose veins.

TREATMENT

All expectant mothers should practice good prenatal care, including a nutritious diet and regular exercise and keeping all appointments with the obstetrician for checkups and testing as needed. Even with the best of care, complications can arise. Pregnant women who experience any of these danger signals should seek immediate medical help: severe persistent abdominal pain; vaginal bleeding (light spotting or staining in the first half of pregnancy may not be an emergency, but bleeding that occurs later in the pregnancy is); blurry vision; swelling of the face, eyelids, or fingers; fever and chills; severe persistent headache (especially during the last trimester); or rupture of the amniotic sac (breaking of the waters).

SELF-HELP AND COMPLEMENTARY CARE

Although pregnancy can be a time of great joy, the accompanying physical discomfort and emotional stress can take their toll. Complementary therapies can provide a great deal of relief during pregnancy. Before including any of these or other complementary therapies in your life, talk to your physician.

- **Stress reduction activities.** Meditation, breathing awareness, self-hypnosis, visualization, and relaxation exercises can provide relief from physical discomfort.

- **Massage.** Look for a therapist who specializes in treatment for pregnant women. Some communities and massage centers offer special sessions for pregnant women. Massage can be helpful for lower back pain, hormonal headaches, leg cramps, and other discomforts associated with pregnancy.

- **Acupuncture.** Look for a qualified practitioner who has experience working with pregnant women. Acupuncture can be helpful for symptoms of pregnancy, including lower back pain, headache, varicose veins, nausea, and edema.

READ MORE ABOUT IT

Magee, Susan, and Kara Nakisbendi. *The Pregnancy Countdown Book: Nine Months of Practical Tips, Useful Advice, and Uncensored Truths.* Quirk Books, 2006.

Mayo Clinic. *Mayo Clinic Guide to a Healthy Pregnancy.* Collins, 2004.

Murkoff, Heidi, and Sharon Mazel. *What to Expect When You're Expecting.* 4th ed. Workman Publishing Company, 2008.

PREMATURE OVARIAN FAILURE (POF)

About 1 percent of women in the United States have premature ovarian failure (POF), which is the loss of normal function of the ovaries before age forty. Although POF is sometimes called premature menopause, POF is somewhat different from premature menopause. Women with premature menopause stop having periods, but some women with POF continue to have sporadic periods for years and may even become pregnant. Hot flashes, sleep problems, mood swings, vaginal dryness, low sex drive, painful sex, bladder control problems, and night sweats are also possible symptoms.

CAUSES AND RISK FACTORS

It appears that your risk of developing POF increases with age: by age thirty-five your risk is about 1 in 250; by age forty, it's 1 in 100. Family history also is a risk factor: about 10 percent of cases of POF are familial.

For most women with POF, the cause of their condition is unknown. What researchers do know is that the ovaries hold thousands of immature follicles, which contain eggs. At the beginning of each menstrual cycle, the pituitary gland secretes follicle-stimulating hormone (FSH). This hormone causes some follicles to begin maturing and also to make estrogen. As estrogen levels rise they signal the pituitary gland that FSH is no longer needed. If the follicles don't mature properly and release estrogen, the level of follicle-stimulating hormone will continue to increase and remain high.

When ovarian function is normal, the pituitary gland then releases another hormone, called luteinizing hormone (LH). This hormone causes the mature follicle to open and release the egg, resulting in ovulation. In POF, however, without the estrogen released by maturing follicles and the subsequent rise in luteinizing hormone, ovulation doesn't occur.

DIAGNOSIS

Along with your medical history, signs and symptoms, any history of exposure to toxins such as chemotherapy or radiation therapy, and information about your periods, your doctor will need to order several blood tests to help with the diagnosis.

- **Follicle-stimulating hormone (FSH) test.** Women with POF often have very high levels of FSH in their blood. Normal FSH levels are 10–15 mIU/ml, for example, while women with POF often have levels greater than 40 mIU/ml.

- **Karyotype.** Some women with POF may have only one X chromosome instead of two or may have another type of chromosomal defect.

- **Luteinizing hormone (LH) test.** Women with POF usually have LH levels that are lower than their FSH levels.

- **Pregnancy test.** This rules out an unexpected pregnancy.

- **Serum estradiol test.** A low level of this type of estrogen is an indication of POF.

PREVENTION AND TREATMENT

Generally, POF is treated with estrogen and progesterone to help prevent osteoporosis and to relieve the symptoms of estrogen deficiency. Treatment can be in the form of a pill or a patch and typically is recommended until a woman reaches the average age of natural menopause, which is around fifty to fifty-four. Supplementation with calcium and vitamin D also is recommended to protect bone health and the risk of developing osteoporosis because of the lack of estrogen.

Concerns about taking hormone replacement therapy because of its association with breast cancer and cardiovascular disease should be discussed with your physician. However, many experts believe that the benefits of hormone replacement in women with POF far outweigh the possible risks.

SELF-HELP AND COMPLEMENTARY CARE
Infertility is a common consequence of POF, and for women who still want to have children, this can be devastating. Although a very small percentage of women with POF do become pregnant, experts do not know which women will be able to achieve natural pregnancy. If you want children and have POF, you can talk to your physician about in vitro fertilization, or you may want to consider adoption.

OTHER HELPFUL INFORMATION
Very low estrogen levels combined with the stress associated with infertility and other health complications of POF may cause you to become depressed or anxious. It is important to recognize this possibility and to take steps to ward it off or treat it. One potential source of help is to join a self-help group for women with POF (see the Appendix).

Women with POF are also at increased risk of developing Addison's disease. This disorder occurs when the adrenal glands don't produce enough of certain hormones that are necessary for body functions. It can be fatal if not treated.

READ MORE ABOUT IT
Banerd, Karin. *Menopause Before 40: Coping with Premature Ovarian Failure.* Your Health Press, 2004.

POF Support Group. *Faces of POF: Learning and Living with Premature Ovarian Failure.* International POF Support Group, 2004.

Schover LR. Premature ovarian failure and its consequences: vasomotor symptoms, sexuality, and fertility. *J Clin Oncol* 2008 Feb 10; 26(5): 753–58.

PREMENSTRUAL SYNDROME (PMS)

Some experts say that premenstrual syndrome (PMS) is associated with about 150 different signs and symptoms, and some women with PMS may argue that they have experienced all of them at least one time or another. The possibility of having such a range of signs and symptoms is one thing that makes it difficult to identify PMS. Yet an estimated 75 to 80 percent of menstruating women experience physical and emotional changes every month or most months in the few days before their period starts.

While room does not permit us to list all 150 signs and symptoms, the more common symptoms of PMS include mood swings, tender breasts, food cravings, headache, fatigue, irritability, depression, and water retention. These and other problems are more likely to affect women between their late twenties and early forties.

CAUSES AND RISK FACTORS

The exact causes of PMS are not known, but several factors contribute to it. Hormone changes are the most obvious factor, especially since the signs and symptoms of the condition change as hormone levels fluctuate and they also disappear with pregnancy and menopause. Another factor is brain chemicals, especially serotonin, a neurotransmitter that plays a crucial role in mood. Inadequate levels of serotonin may contribute to premenstrual depression, fatigue, food cravings, and sleep problems.

Some PMS symptoms may be associated with low levels of various important nutrients, including calcium and magnesium. Some research indicates that eating salty foods and drinking caffeinated beverages and alcohol may play a part as well. Stress also is believed to be an aggravating factor, although not a cause of PMS symptoms.

DIAGNOSIS
No test has yet been developed that can positively diagnose premenstrual syndrome, and the condition does not have any unique features that would make diagnosis easy. You can, however, keep a record of your signs and symptoms over the span of two or three menstrual cycles, noting when symptoms first appear, their severity, and when they end, as well as when your period starts and ends. This information can help your physician determine whether you may need testing or further evaluation.

PREVENTION AND TREATMENT
At this point, there are no known ways to prevent premenstrual syndrome, but you can do much to alleviate symptoms. Some conventional medical options are:

- **Antidepressants.** The selective serotonin reuptake inhibitors (SSRIs), which include fluoxetine (Prozac), paroxetine (Paxil), and sertraline (Zoloft), among others, can do more than relieve depression; they may also reduce fatigue, sleep difficulties, and food cravings. Some women find that they need to take these medications daily, while others get relief if they take them only during the two weeks before menstruation begins. This is an option you can discuss with your physician.

- **Nonsteroidal anti-inflammatory drugs (NSAIDs).** Cramping and breast tenderness can be reduced or eliminated if you take these drugs (e.g., ibuprofen, naproxen sodium) before or at the beginning of your period.

- **Oral contraceptives.** One advantage of taking prescription contraceptives is that they stabilize fluctuations in hormone levels and thus offer relief from PMS symptoms. A type of birth control pill that contains the progestin drospirenone along with ethinyl estradiol appears to be more effective than regular birth control pills in reducing the physical and emotional symptoms of PMS.

- **Diuretics.** If attempts to reduce bloating, weight gain, and water retention using nonmedical means do not work (see "Self-Help and Complementary Care"), you may consider a diuretic. Spironolactone can help ease some of these PMS symptoms.

- **Medroxyprogesterone acetate.** If you are experiencing severe PMS symptoms, your doctor can prescribe an injection of medroxyprogesterone acetate, which will temporarily stop ovulation. This option comes with side effects, however, as it may cause weight gain, headache, depressed mood, and increased appetite.

SELF-HELP AND COMPLEMENTARY CARE
Changes to your diet and exercise can have a significant positive impact on PMS symptoms, and without the possibility of side effects from drugs. Consider these suggestions and see how they work for you:

- **Eat more frequent but smaller meals** to help reduce bloating.

- **Limit the amount of salt** and salty foods you eat to reduce fluid retention and bloating. This is an opportunity to try new seasonings and flavorings for your food—for example, fresh garlic; dried or fresh herbs such as basil, thyme, sage, and coriander; or fresh lemon and lime.

- **Avoid caffeine and alcohol.**

- **Choose foods high in complex carbohydrates,** such as vegetables, whole grains, nuts, and fruits.

- **Include foods high in calcium** in your diet every day. These do not need to be dairy foods; greens such as bok choy and broccoli and calcium-fortified soy foods such as tofu, soy beverages, and tempeh provide calcium as well.

- **Exercise.** Spend about thirty minutes per day doing aerobic exercise, such as walking, biking, dancing, tennis, or swimming, which can reduce fatigue and depression.

- **Rest.** Take catnaps (twenty minutes) during the day when possible to help boost your energy and mood.

- **Reduce stress** using techniques that work for you. For some women this includes yoga, tai chi, deep breathing therapy, progressive relaxation exercises, self-hypnosis, visualization, or meditation.

Supplements can also have a positive impact on PMS symptoms. The following supplements have proven useful for many women:

- **Calcium.** A total of 1,200 mg of calcium from both your diet and supplements is suggested. Many experts recommend calcium citrate over other types of cal-cium supplements because it is more bioavailable. If you take a calcium supplement, take no more than 500 mg at one time. Calcium can be taken with food to help reduce the risk of bloating and constipation.

- **Magnesium.** Take 400 mg daily to help reduce breast tenderness, bloating, and fluid retention.

- **Vitamin B$_6$.** A daily dose of 50 to 100 mg may help with a variety of PMS symptoms.

- **Vitamin E.** This vitamin helps reduce the production of prostaglandins, which can cause cramps and breast tenderness. A suggested dose is 400 IU daily.

OTHER HELPFUL INFORMATION
Although the scientific evidence does not always support the use of herbs for PMS symptoms, there are many anecdotal reports of their effectiveness. Some of the herbs that have been helpful include the following:

- **Black cohosh** helps with sleep problems, hot flashes, headache, and depressive mood. The suggested dose is 80 mg of extract (standardized to 2.5 percent total triterpenes) in capsule form once or twice daily, or 250 mg once daily.

- **Chasteberry** helps with cramping. Take 10 drops of tincture in water every morning.

- **Ginger** is helpful for nausea and fatigue. Drink one cup of ginger tea daily.

- **Dandelion** is a natural diuretic. It helps reduce bloating, water retention, weight gain, and breast tenderness. Drink one to three cups of dandelion tea daily. Take along with chasteberry for a synergistic effect.

- **Evening primrose oil** helps eliminate symptoms associated with inflammation, such as breast tenderness and cramping. The suggested dose is 250 to 500 mg daily in capsule form.

Deborah Mitchell

READ MORE ABOUT IT

Glenville, Marilyn. *Overcoming PMS the Natural Way.* Piatkus Books, 2006.

Jones, Andrew. *The All Natural Cure to Your PMS.* 48 Hour Books, 2007.

Redmond, Geoffrey. *The Hormonally Vulnerable Woman.* Collins, 2004.

PROLAPSED BLADDER (CYSTOCELE)

Prolapsed bladder or dropped bladder, also known as cysto-cele, occurs when the wall between a woman's bladder and vagina weakens and stretches, which allows the bladder to bulge into the vagina. It is the most common type of pelvic organ prolapse, a phrase that refers to the descent (prolapse) of the walls of the vagina and/or uterus below their normal positions. The muscles, ligaments, and connective tissue in and around the vagina support the pelvic organs, but when this system weakens, the pelvic organs slip out of place.

Symptoms of cystocele may include a feeling of fullness or pressure in your vagina or pelvis, especially when you have been standing for a long time; a feeling that you haven't com-pletely emptied your bladder after urinating; increased dis-comfort when you lift, strain, or cough; recurrent bladder infections; urinary stress incontinence when you laugh, cough, or sneeze; and pain or urinary leakage during sexual inter-course. If other organs also move into the region in front of the vagina, the condition is called an anterior prolapse.

CAUSES AND RISK FACTORS
The most common causes of cystocele are pregnancy and childbirth, both of which stretch and weaken the muscles and ligaments that support the vagina. Your risk of developing cystocele increases:

- **With age.** Muscle and nerve function decline naturally as you age, and especially after menopause, when pelvic muscles weaken with the dramatic decrease in estrogen levels.

- **With excessive straining.** Chronic constipation or heavy lifting can increase your risk.

- **After childbirth.** Women who have had one or more children delivered vaginally have a greater risk of cystocele.

- **After hysterectomy.** Removal of the uterus may contribute to a weakened pelvic floor.

For some women, genetics play a role, as they have a natural tendency for weak connective tissues in the pelvic region.

DIAGNOSIS

Your doctor will conduct a pelvic examination to determine if you have cystocele. During the examination, he or she will attempt to feel if there is a bulge in your vaginal wall. You may also be asked to bear down as if you were having a bowel movement and/or to contract the muscles of your pelvis (as if you were trying to stop urinating) to check the strength of your pelvic floor muscles. Your health care provider will likely give your cystocele a "grade": grade 1 is when the bladder drops only a short way into the vagina; grade 2 is when the bladder sinks to the vaginal opening; and grade 3 is defined as when the bladder bulges through the vaginal opening.

PREVENTION AND TREATMENT

Squeeze, hold, release, and repeat: one way to help prevent cystocele is to do Kegel exercises, which strengthen the pelvic floor muscles (see "Kegel Exercises" in Part II). Other preventive measures: eat a high-fiber diet to avoid constipation, lift using your legs instead of your back, avoid heavy lifting, don't smoke, treat chronic cough or bronchitis, and maintain a healthy weight.

Treatment of cystocele depends on how severe it is. If you have few or no obvious symptoms, your doctor may suggest you regularly do Kegel exercises and follow other preventive measures. If more aggressive action is needed, he or she may ˙ recommend a vaginal pessary, which can support the bladder (see "Pessary" in Part II). In some cases, a vaginal diaphragm or large tampon can be used instead of a pessary. A pessary is usually a temporary alternative to surgery, although some women use a pessary for many years.

If the cystocele is very uncomfortable, you may want to consider surgery. In most cases, a surgeon returns the prolapse to its proper place and tightens the ligaments and muscles of the pelvic floor. Cystocele may recur, however, partly because pelvic muscles continue to weaken with age. Although surgery can be repeated, results the second time around typically are not as effective. If you have a prolapsed uterus as well as cystocele, your doctor may recommend removing your uterus (hysterectomy).

SELF-HELP AND COMPLEMENTARY CARE
Kegel exercises are a popular way to treat yourself if you have cystocele, and you can enhance those exercises by using biofeedback. A biofeedback therapist can help you learn how to contract the proper muscles so you can get the maximum benefit from these exercises.

OTHER HELPFUL INFORMATION
If you have a large cystocele, it is suggested that you avoid surgical correction until you are done having children. If the cystocele is severe and you need surgery, you can still have children, although your doctor will likely recommend you have a cesarean delivery.

READ MORE ABOUT IT
Glazer HI, Laine CD. Pelvic floor muscle biofeedback in the treatment of urinary incontinence: a literature review. *Appl Psychophysiol Biofeedback* 2006 Sep; 31(3): 187–201.

Deborah Mitchell

Hulme, Janet A. *Beyond Kegel: Fabulous Four Exercises and More to Prevent and Treat Incontinence.* 2nd ed. Phoenix Publishing, 2002.

Klutke CG. Female pelvic prolapse. *Mo Med* 2007 Sep–Oct; 104(5): 430–34.

PROLAPSED UTERUS

Prolapsed uterus, or uterine prolapse, occurs when the uterus drops from its normal position in the pelvic cavity and falls into or outside the vagina. It is a progressive condition that gets worse over time if not treated. The first degree of uterine prolapse is when the cervix droops into the vagina. This progresses to the cervix sticking to the opening of the vagina. The third degree is when the cervix is outside the vagina, while the most serious form of uterine prolapse is when the entire uterus is outside the vagina. This last condition is also called procidentia.

A prolapsed uterus is most often seen among postmenopausal women, but it can also occur in younger women. Other conditions are often associated with prolapsed uterus, as they also weaken the muscles that help support the uterus. Those conditions include bulging of the bladder into the vagina (see "Prolapsed Bladder," herniation of the small bowel into the vagina (called enterocele), and bulging of the recum into the vagina (called rectocele).

CAUSES AND RISK FACTORS

The uterus is held in place inside the pelvis with the help of various muscles, ligaments, and tissues. Events such as childbirth, difficult labor and delivery, chronic coughing and/or chronic pulmonary disease, obesity, chronic constipation, and the natural loss of estrogen as women age can all weaken the supporting muscles, causing the uterus to collapse into the vaginal canal.

DIAGNOSIS

To diagnose uterine prolapse, your doctor will likely ask about your sexual history and your symptoms, which may include a feeling of fullness in your vagina, bladder control problems, increased vaginal discharge, a dragging feeling in your lower abdomen and back, increased urinary frequency, and a reduction in symptoms when you lie down. He or she will also do a pelvic examination to feel for the prolapse and perhaps even order an ultrasound or magnetic resonance imaging (MRI) to verify the diagnosis and the extent of the prolapse.

PREVENTION AND TREATMENT

Prevention of uterine prolapse is largely limited to trying to tone and strengthen the muscles that help support the uterus. The most common exercises for this purpose are called Kegel exercises, which can be performed anytime, anywhere (see "Kegel Exercises" in Part II). Although they can improve the muscle tone in the pelvic floor and help stress-related urinary incontinence, they cannot repair any damage that has been done. Another precaution is to avoid heavy lifting.

Hysterectomy is often viewed as *the* treatment for women who are experiencing significant symptoms because of a prolapsed uterus, but there are other options you can discuss with your physician. One is use of a pessary (see "Pessary" in Part II), a rubber, plastic, or silicone-based device that is placed into the vagina to help support the uterus. Another option is called a uterine suspension, a surgical procedure that involves shortening the ligament that supports the uterus. This procedure can be done via a laparoscope and has a fairly good success rate.

If neither of these options provides the relief you need, then a hysterectomy may be an option unless you want to have children. If having children is not an issue but you don't want to go into menopause, then a hysterectomy without removing your ovaries may be for you.

SELF-HELP AND COMPLEMENTARY CARE
Daily Kegel exercises are a great self-help step for uterine prolapse, but you can also consider these tips:

- If you are overweight, work toward a healthy weight.

- Eat high-fiber foods that will help you avoid constipation and thus the need to strain.

- Avoid wearing any clothing that is tight around your abdomen, including girdles or tight pants.

- Avoid frequent heavy lifting.

READ MORE ABOUT IT
Brown JS et al. Pelvic organ prolapse surgery in the United States, 1997. *Am J Obstetr Gynecol* 2002; 186:712–16.

Scott RJ, Lazarou G. Abdominal approaches to uterine suspension. In Gersherson DM, ed. *Operative Techniques in Gynecologic Surgery*. Philadelphia: WB Saunders Co, 2000.

RETROVERTED UTERUS

A retroverted uterus, also called a tipped uterus, is a condition in which the uterus is tipped back toward the back of the pelvis. It occurs in 25 to 30 percent of women, but since many of them have only minor symptoms or none at all, they often do not even know they have it. The main symptoms of a tipped uterus include pain during intercourse or pain during menstruation, but you may also experience back pain during intercourse, urinary tract infections, difficulty using tampons, minor urinary incontinence, and fertility problems.

CAUSES AND RISK FACTORS
A retroverted uterus can develop for several reasons:

- The uterus may not move into a forward position as it should as you mature.

- Childbirth can cause the uterus to tip forward or backward. Although the uterus returns to a forward position after childbirth in most cases, for some women the ligaments that hold the uterus stretch or lose their tension during pregnancy and do not regain it, causing the uterus to tip.

- Scars from endometriosis, salpingitis, pelvic inflammatory disease, or fibroids can cause the uterus to shift to a tilted position.

DIAGNOSIS

A tipped uterus can be detected during a pelvic examination. If you have any reason to think you may have a tipped uterus, ask your doctor to examine you.

PREVENTION AND TREATMENT

There's no way to prevent a tipped uterus, but there are several options for treatment. One of two nonsurgical approaches includes an exercise called "knee-chest," which may help reposition a tipped uterus temporarily. This exercise is not effective if your uterus is tipped because of endometriosis, fibroids, or pelvic infections. Your health care professional can show you how to do this exercise.

Another option is a pessary, a plastic, rubber, or silicone device that you place inside your vagina to help support a tipped uterus. This is considered a temporary solution for relief of pelvic pain.

A surgical solution is called uterine suspension, which repositions the uterus from a backward-facing position to a forward-facing one. A newer version of this procedure is called the UPLIFT procedure, and it has fewer postoperative complications than the older option. The UPLIFT procedure involves shortening and strengthening the ligaments that hold the uterus so that it falls back into a more normal position. This procedure can provide lasting relief from painful sex for most women and from painful menstruation for some.

OTHER HELPFUL INFORMATION

If you have a tipped uterus and wonder if it will affect your ability to become or stay pregnant, the answer is that it most likely will not. In most cases, a tipped uterus is not a cause of infertility. If your doctor has exhausted all other possibilities, a fertility specialist may suggest you undergo surgery to correct the position of your uterus. If you are already pregnant, by the time you reach weeks ten to twelve, your uterus will no longer be tipped. In very rare cases, the uterus does not move into the proper position at this point, in which case a miscarriage is possible.

READ MORE ABOUT IT

Haylen BT. The retroverted uterus: ignored to date but core to prolapse. *Int Uregynecol J Pelvic Floor Dysfunct* 2006 Nov; 17(6): 555–58.

Haylen BT et al. A standardized ultrasonic diagnosis and an accurate prevalence for the retroverted uterus in general gynaecology patients. *Aust N Z J Obstet Gynaecol* 2007 Aug; 47(4): 326–28.

SEXUAL DYSFUNCTION

If your interest in sex has vanished or your body just doesn't respond the way it used to, or if you have recurrent problems with sexual response, you're feeling upset about it, and it's affecting your relationship with your partner, you're not alone. Approximately 40 percent of women experience sexual dysfunction at some point in their lifetime.

Sexual dysfunction in women can develop at any age, but the problems seem to be most common when their hormones are in transition—for example, among women who have just had a baby or those who are entering menopause. Your problems with sex might be classified as female sexual dysfunction if one or more of the following issues are upsetting you:

- Your sexual desire is low or absent.

- You can't maintain arousal during sexual activity, or you don't become aroused even though you want to have sex.

- You cannot experience an orgasm.

- Sexual intercourse is painful.

CAUSES AND RISK FACTORS
Sexual difficulties can be caused by physical, hormonal, psychological, and/or social factors.

- **Physical.** Certain physical conditions may cause or contribute to sexual problems, including arthritis, fatigue, headache/migraine, neurological disorders (e.g., multiple sclerosis), urinary or bowel problems, and chronic pain disorders. Some medical treatments are known to reduce sex drive and the ability to achieve orgasm, including some antidepressants, blood pressure medications, antihistamines, and chemotherapy.

- **Hormonal.** A woman's hormones seem to be in constant flux, but there are times when they are especially changeable in ways that can have an impact on sexual desire and pleasure. After childbirth and during breast-feeding, for example, changes in hormones can cause vaginal dryness and have an effect on your desire to have sex. During the transition to menopause, estrogen levels begin to decline, which can result in changes in sexual responsiveness and in the health of genital tissues. The clitoris, for example, is more exposed as the skin around it becomes thinner, and this additional exposure may cause unpleasant sensations. The vaginal lining also becomes thinner and less elastic and requires more stimulation to lubricate. These changes can result in painful intercourse and difficulty achieving orgasm.

- **Psychological/social.** Stress, anxiety, and depression can all cause or contribute to sexual dysfunction, as can problems with body image, religious and cultural issues, the demands of new motherhood, and relationship conflicts with your mate.

DIAGNOSIS

If you are having sexual problems and would like to get a diagnosis, you will need to be forthcoming with your physician. He or she will need to know about your sexual history and your current concerns. You will also need a pelvic exam so your doctor can note if there are any physical changes that may be responsible for your lack of sexual enjoyment.

Female sexual dysfunction is usually divided into four categories, which have some overlap:

- **Low sexual desire.** You have little or no sex drive.

- **Sexual arousal disorder.** You may have a strong desire for sex, but you have problems or are not able to become aroused or maintain arousal.

- **Orgasmic disorder.** Despite sufficient, ongoing stimulation, you have continuing difficulty achieving orgasm.

- **Sexual pain disorder.** Sexual stimulation and/or vaginal contact are painful for you.

PREVENTION AND TREATMENT

Female sexual dysfunction usually involves both physical and emotional factors, so both should be addressed in treatment. In many cases, behavioral therapy, such as couples therapy, stress management, and individual counseling, can be very helpful for both the woman and her partner. Here are some noninvasive, nonmedical tips to treat female sexual dysfunction:

- **Avoid excessive alcohol.** Too much alcohol can hinder your sexual responsiveness.

- **Engage in regular aerobic exercise.** The plusses include elevated mood, improved body image, and better stamina.

- **Communicate openly.** You and your partner should practice talking openly and honestly about sex, your likes and dislikes, and your feelings. This type of communication can make a significant positive difference in your sexual satisfaction.

- **Strengthen the pelvic muscles.** Exercises to strengthen the pelvic floor muscles (see "Kegel Exercises" in Part II) can help with sexual arousal and orgasm problems.

- **Consider counseling.** A counselor or therapist who specializes in relationship and sexual problems may help you better understand your sexual identity and needs, learn how to cope with or overcome any fears and anxiety about sex and intimacy, and work on communication skills. These sessions can be done alone and/or with your partner.

- **Explore underlying medical conditions.** Frequently there is an underlying medical or hormonal problem that affects sexuality. Depending on what your current medical condition is, your physician may need to adjust any medications you are taking (including any drugs for depression), treat any thyroid or hormonal problems, and consider ways to treat any significant pelvic pain or other pain that is affecting sexuality.

- **Try hormone therapy.** If your sexual dysfunction is associated with hormone fluctuations or imbalance, then various types of hormone therapy may help. However, hormone therapies will not correct sexual difficulties that are not caused by hormones and that have unresolved psychological/ emotional causes.

  - **Estrogen therapy** can improve vaginal tone and elasticity, enhance vaginal blood flow, improve lubrication, and have a positive effect on mood.

  - **Progestin therapy,** when taken with estrogen, resulted in improved sexual arousal and desire in some studies. Since progestin is usually given to balance the effect of estrogen and not to treat female sexual dysfunction, this possible benefit from progestin is under investigation.

- **Testosterone therapy** has been helpful for some women who have low levels of the hormone and have sexual dysfunction, but not all studies have shown a benefit. Testosterone use in women has side effects, such as acne, enlargement of the clitoris, mood changes, and growth of excess body hair on the face and chest. Use of testosterone should be carefully monitored by your doctor should you choose to try it.

READ MORE ABOUT IT

Hall, Kathryn. *Reclaiming Your Sexual Self: How You Can Bring Desire Back into Your Life.* Wiley, 2004.

Keesling, Barbara. *Sexual Healing: The Complete Guide to Overcoming Common Sexual Problems.* Hunter House, 2006.

Schnarch, David, and James Maddock. *Resurrecting Sex: Solving Sexual Problems and Revolutionizing Your Relationship.* Harper Paperbacks, 2003.

SYPHILIS

Syphilis is a sexually transmitted disease (STD) that affects the genitals, skin, and mucous membranes, but it may also attack other parts of the body, including the heart and brain. If it is not treated promptly, it can cause serious complications, including death, but early treatment can successfully eliminate the disease.

The signs and symptoms of syphilis occur in four stages:

- **Primary.** These signs may occur from ten days to three months after exposure. They include small, painless sores on the body part where the infection was transmitted, usually the genitals, lips, tongue, or rectum. These signs typically disappear without treatment, but the disease is still present and may reappear in the secondary or tertiary stage.

- **Secondary.** These signs and symptoms may begin two to ten weeks after the sore(s) appeared and may include:

  - Rash accompanied by red or red-brown penny-sized sores over your body, including your soles and palms

  - Fever

- Soreness and aching muscles

- Fatigue

These signs and symptoms may disappear within a few weeks or return again and again for as long as one year.

- **Latent.** No symptoms are present during this stage, which follows the secondary stage in some people. Signs and symptoms may never come back, or the disease may move on to the tertiary stage.

- **Tertiary.** If syphilis is not treated, the bacteria may spread and cause serious internal organ damage and death. Some signs and symptoms of tertiary syphilis are:

    - Neurological problems, such as stroke, poor muscle coordination, numbness, paralysis, visual and hearing problems, dementia, personality changes, and meningitis

    - Cardiovascular problems, including aneurysm, inflammation of the aorta and other blood vessels, and valvular heart disease

CAUSES AND RISK FACTORS

Syphilis can be spread during unprotected vaginal, oral, or anal sex through contact with an open sore or a skin rash. It cannot be spread through contact with doorknobs, swimming pools, hot tubs, toilet seats, or shared clothing. The bacteria (*Treponema pallidum*) enter the body through the vagina, mouth, penis, anus, or broken skin. Because the bacteria are extremely sensitive to light, temperature changes, and air, intimate sexual contact is the way virtually all cases of syphilis are spread, except when an infected mother passes it along to her child during delivery.

DIAGNOSIS

If you have painless sores in your genital area, see your doctor. To make a diagnosis, he or she may collect a sample of cells from a sore, or you may provide a blood sample that can be checked for the presence of antibodies to the bacteria that cause the disease.

PREVENTION AND TREATMENT

The best way to reduce your risk of syphilis is to:

- Abstain from sex

- Limit your sexual activity to a single, uninfected partner

- Use a latex condom if you don't know the STD status of your partner

Early diagnosis and treatment with an antibiotic can eliminate the organism that causes syphilis and stop progression of the disease. The usual treatment is penicillin or tetracycline, and the amount prescribed depends on the stage of syphilis you are in. The first day you take your antibiotic you may experience the Jarisch-Herxheimer reaction, which includes fever, chills, achy pain, headache, and nausea. This reaction typically lasts only one day and is believed to be the body's reaction to so many bacteria dying at once.

OTHER HELPFUL INFORMATION

If you have syphilis and are pregnant, you may pass along the infection to your unborn child, because the bacteria travel in the bloodstream through the placenta. More than half the women who are pregnant and who have active untreated syphilis infect their babies, and nearly half the babies who contract syphilis die. Babies born with syphilis who are not treated early may develop swollen joints, bone pain and abnormalities, hearing and vision problems, disfigured teeth, and death.

READ MORE ABOUT IT
Daskalakis D. Syphilis: continuing public health and diagnostic challenges. *Curr HIV/AIDS Rep* 2008 May; 5(2): 72–77.

Hayden, Deborah. *Pox: Genius, Madness and the Mysteries of Syphilis.* Basic Books, 2003.

Stokes, John H. *The Third Great Plague: A Discussion of Syphilis for Everyday People.* BiblioBazaar, 2006.

TRICHOMONIASIS

Every year, an estimated 7.4 million new cases of trichomoniasis occur in women and men. Trichomoniasis is the most common curable sexually transmitted disease in young, sexually active women, and the vagina is the most common site of infection. Signs and symptoms include a frothy, yellow-green vaginal discharge that has a strong odor, discomfort during intercourse and urination, itching of the genital area, and, in rare cases, lower abdominal pain. Symptoms typically appear within five to twenty-eight days of exposure.

CAUSES AND RISK FACTORS

As with other sexually transmitted diseases, the main risk factor for trichomoniasis is having unprotected sex. A one-celled organism called *Trichomonas vaginalis* is the culprit behind trichomoniasis. The organisms can survive for several hours at room temperature on moist surfaces and objects and so can be transmitted on clothing, bedding, towels, or toilet seats by an infected woman.

DIAGNOSIS

Trichomoniasis can be diagnosed by a health care professional who does a physical examination and a blood test to identify the offending parasite. Women who have trichomoniasis may have a telltale sign of small red sores on the vaginal wall or cervix.

PREVENTION AND TREATMENT

To avoid transmission of this sexually transmitted disease, you can:

- Abstain from sexual contact

- Limit your sexual activities to a long-term mutually monogamous relationship with a partner known to be free of infection

- Always use a latex condom with partners whose infection status is not known

The prescription drugs metronidazole and tinidazole are both effective in curing trichomoniasis. Metronidazole can be used if you are pregnant. If you are being treated for trichomoniasis, you should abstain from sex until you and your partner have completed treatment and have no symptoms. Having trichomoniasis once and successfully treating it does not protect you from getting it again.

SELF-HELP AND COMPLEMENTARY CARE

Some women have tried using herbs to relieve symptoms along with conventional drug treatment. One approach is to make a garlic suppository by peeling a clove of garlic, wrapping it in gauze, securing a string in the wrapping so you can easily remove the suppository, and inserting it overnight into your vagina like a tampon. You can dip the suppository into vegetable oil to make it easier to insert. Garlic, which is a potent antimicrobial, can help relieve irritation. Another option is to prepare a douche with a mixture of myrrh (*Commiphora myrrha)* and goldenseal (*Hydrastis canadensis)*, 1/2 teaspoon each of dried herb steeped in 16 ounces of hot water for five minutes. Strain out the herbs and allow the mixture to cool before using twice a day for one to two weeks.

OTHER HELPFUL INFORMATION

If you are pregnant and have trichomoniasis, it can cause your baby to be born early or to have a very low birth weight (less than five pounds). The Centers for Disease Control and Prevention recommend that women with the disease who have symptoms should be treated, but women without symptoms do not need treatment. Metronidazole appears to be safe for pregnant women, but many experts recommend that women not take it during their first trimester because it may harm the baby. After the end of the first trimester, metronidazole is considered to be safe.

Having trichomoniasis may increase your risk of infection with HIV, and it also may increase the rate of infection or reactivation with human papillomavirus. Trichomoniasis also commonly occurs along with other STDs, especially gonorrhea.

READ MORE ABOUT IT

Sutton M et al. The prevalence of Trichomonas vaginalis infection among reproductive-age women in the United States 2001–2004. *Clin Infect Dis* 2007 Nov 15; 45(1): 1319–26.

Verteramo R et al. Trichomonas vaginalis infection: Risk indicators among women attending for routine gynecologic examination. *J Obstet Gynaecol Res* 2008 Apr; 34(2): 233–37.

UNUSUAL LACTATION (GALACTORRHEA)

Galactorrhea (unusual or inappropriate lactation) is a condition in which a woman's breast makes milk (or the nipples leak milk) even though she is not breast-feeding a baby. One or both breasts may make milk and the breast may leak either with stimulation or without being touched. Along with the milk flow, women often also experience headache, vision problems, irregular or cessation of periods, acne, an increase in hair growth on the chest or chin, and a loss of interest in sex. Approximately 20 to 25 percent of women experience galactorrhea at some point in their lives.

CAUSES AND RISK FACTORS
Lactation requires estrogen, progesterone, and especially prolactin, the hormone that stimulates milk production. Factors that cause prolactin levels to rise, such as stress, sleep, sexual intercourse, and suckling, may trigger galactorrhea. Other possible causes include hypothyroidism, pituitary adenomas, neurologic disorders, some medications, or an intracranial mass or tumor. Overall, about one-third of galactorrhea cases have an unknown cause, 20 percent are caused by medications or herbs (e.g., antidepressants, antihypertensives, oral contraceptives, opiates; anise, fennel, nettle, red clover), and more than 18 percent are associated with a tumor, adenoma, or similar growth.

DIAGNOSIS
Your doctor will likely do a blood test to see if you are pregnant and to determine your hormone levels, especially of prolactin. Other tests may include thyroid and renal function tests and a magnetic resonance image (MRI) of the brain.

PREVENTION AND TREATMENT
Often, galactorrhea goes away on its own over time, and so no treatment is necessary. If there is an underlying cause such as a tumor, hypothyroidism, or a neurologic condition, appropriate treatment of the condition should eliminate galactorrhea.

If no specific cause can be found for galactorrhea and the milk discharge is embarrassing or troublesome, certain medications can reduce prolactin levels in the body and may eliminate galactorrhea, including bromocriptine and cabergoline.

SELF-HELP AND COMPLEMENTARY CARE
In many cases, time is the only treatment for galactorrhea. While you are waiting for galactorrhea to resolve itself, you can help it along by avoiding stimulation of your breasts during sexual activity, by wearing clothing that does not rub or irritate your breasts, and by minimizing breast self-examination to no more than once per month.

OTHER HELPFUL INFORMATION
High levels of prolactin (hyperprolactinemia) can, over time, reduce bone density and thus increase the risk of osteoporosis. Use of dopamine agonists (e.g., bromocritine, cabergoline) can reduce prolactin levels and your risk of bone loss.

READ MORE ABOUT IT
Molitch ME. Drugs and prolactin. *Pituitary* 2008 Apr 11.

Pena KS, Rosenfeld J. Evaluation and treatment of galactorrhea. *Am Fam Physician* 2001; 63: 1763–70.

URINARY INCONTINENCE

Millions of women of all ages sometimes experience urinary incontinence, which is an involuntary loss of urine. This medical condition is twice as common among women as men. Some women lose only a few drops when they cough or sneeze, while others feel an urgent need to urinate just before they lose control of a large amount of urine. Many women experience both of these symptoms from time to time. The uncertainty of not knowing when incontinence will occur can be very stressful and, in some cases, makes women afraid to participate in many activities or to socialize for fear of embarrassing themselves. The involuntary release of urine during sexual activity, for example, can make women avoid sex altogether.

There are several types of urinary incontinence. *Stress incontinence* occurs when laughing, coughing, sneezing, or other physical movements put pressure on the bladder, causing you to leak urine. *Urge incontinence* is a sudden and unexplainable urge to urinate. Some women get the urge when they hear water running or when they just touch water; others release urine during sleep or when washing dishes. *Overactive bladder* occurs when abnormal nerves send signals to the bladder at the wrong times, causing its muscles to constrict without warning. Not only does this lead to the need to urinate eight or more times a day and two or more times per night, but also the need is immediate—so urgent and uncontrollable that some women wear special undergarments when they go out to avoid having an accident.

CAUSES AND RISK FACTORS

Incontinence occurs because the muscles and nerves that help control the holding or release of urine have been compromised or are dysfunctional in some way. Although older age can be considered a risk factor, incontinence is not an inevitable part of older age. Pregnancy and childbirth both can weaken the muscles, and the more times you are pregnant and give birth, the greater the risk of urinary incontinence. Menopause also plays a role, as the dramatic decline in estrogen, which helps maintain the lining of the bladder and urethra, means the urethra can't control the release of urine as well. Other causes of urinary incontinence may include stroke, bladder stones, urinary stones, hysterectomy, uncontrolled diabetes, hyperthyroidism, neurologic injury, multiple sclerosis, certain medications (e.g., antidepressants, antihypertensives, diuretics, heart medications, sedatives), and physical problems associated with aging.

DIAGNOSIS

To uncover the cause of your urinary incontinence, your physician will need to know your medical history and about your symptoms. You should also have a complete physical examination, and depending on what your doctor discovers, you may need some tests, including the following:

- **Bladder diary.** You will need to keep a record of how much you drink, when you urinate, the amount of urine you produce, the number of incontinence episodes, and whether you had an urge to urinate. Your urine production can be tracked using a special pan, which your doctor may give you, that fits over your toilet rim and measures output.

- **Blood test.** This may reveal chemicals or other substances that may be causing your incontinence.

- **Urinalysis.** A urine sample can be checked for infections, blood, or other abnormalities.

The following tests may be ordered if the findings to this point are inconclusive:

- **Pelvic ultrasound.** This can be used to look at the entire urinary tract for abnormalities.

- **Stress test.** Your doctor will ask you to cough vigorously or bear down as he or she examines you and looks for loss of urine.

- **Cystogram.** This is an X-ray of the bladder. A special dye is inserted into your urethra and bladder through a catheter, and as you urinate, a series of X-rays can document any problems in the urinary tract.

- **Urodynamic testing.** This test measures the strength of your bladder muscle and urinary sphincter. The test involves placing a catheter into your urethra and bladder and filling your bladder with water while a monitor records the pressure inside your bladder.

- **Cystoscopy.** A cystoscope (thin tube with a tiny lens) is inserted into your urethra, which allows the doctor to look for and remove abnormalities in your urinary tract.

PREVENTION AND TREATMENT

Preventing or reducing the impact of urinary incontinence may be as simple as practicing pelvic floor muscle exercises, especially during pregnancy, although these exercises do not address all of the possible causes of urinary incontinence. Other preventive measures include avoiding bladder irritants (e.g., caffeine, alcohol), maintaining a healthy weight, and eating more fiber to help avoid constipation.

Treatment options fall into four categories: behavioral

techniques, medications, devices, and surgery. Here's a brief overview of possible treatments, beginning with behavioral and lifestyle changes.

- **Pelvic floor muscle exercises.** Also known as Kegel exercises, these can be especially helpful for stress incontinence. It will likely take several months of doing the exercises correctly to notice an improvement. (See "Kegel Exercises" in Part II.)

- **Bladder training.** This technique involves learning to delay urination when you get the urge to go. For example, you may hold off for ten minutes every time you feel an urge to urinate. Over time you will train yourself to increase the hold time to twenty minutes or more.

- **Management of diet and fluids.** Some people only need to make adjustments to their fluid intake—how much and when they consume it—and/or need to reduce or eliminate alcohol or caffeine. Avoiding acidic foods (e.g., meat, dairy products, alcohol, peanuts, chocolate), which can irritate your bladder, also may help.

- **Medications.** Possible choices include antispasmodic drugs (e.g., tolterodine, oxybutynin, darifenacin), imipramine (may be used along with other medications to treat incontinence), and antibiotics (to treat infection).

- **Electrical stimulation.** Electrodes are inserted into your rectum or vagina to stimulate and strengthen your pelvic floor muscles. The electrical stimulation used is very gentle, and it can take several months and many treatments for this approach to work. This option is usually reserved for patients with severe urge incontinence who don't respond to behavioral techniques or medications.

- **Pessary.** This is a stiff ring that is inserted into your vagina to help hold up the bladder (see "Pessary" in Part II).

- **Urethral inserts.** These are tiny plugs that you can insert into your urethra to prevent urine from leaking out. They are available by prescription.

- **Bulking agents.** This treatment involves injecting bulking materials into the tissue that surrounds the urethra, which tightens the seal of the sphincter. The procedure requires minimal anesthesia and takes only about three minutes.

- **Sacral nerve stimulator.** A small device is implanted under the skin in your abdomen, and a wire from the device is connected to a sacral nerve, which is involved in bladder control. The device sends electrical pulses that stimulate the nerve and help control the bladder.

- **Sling procedure.** This is the most common surgery for women with stress incontinence. A surgeon attaches a strip of abdominal tissue, synthetic mesh, or tissue from a donor under the urethra so that it supports and compresses the urethra to prevent leaks. This procedure can be accomplished using various techniques, so you should talk to your surgeon about your options.

- **Bladder neck suspension.** In this procedure, a surgeon makes a 3-to-5-inch incision in the lower abdomen, makes stitches near the neck of the bladder, and secures them to a ligament near the pubic bone or the cartilage of the pubic bone. This technique boosts the urethra and bladder neck. Recovery from this surgery takes about six weeks, and you will need to use a catheter until you can urinate normally.

SELF-HELP AND COMPLEMENTARY CARE

Regular practice of Kegel exercises may be the most helpful step you can take to help prevent and/or treat urinary incontinence. The beauty of these exercises is that they can be done anywhere, at any time, and no one will even know you are doing them; they are free; and there are no side effects. Kegel exercises involve working specific muscles, and like all muscles, if you don't use them, you lose them.

READ MORE ABOUT IT

Minassian VA et al. Urinary incontinence in women: variation in prevalence estimates and risk factors. *Obstet Gynecol* 2008 Feb; 111(2 Pt 1): 324–31.

Hysterectomy may increase risk of urinary incontinence. *Mayo Clin Womens Healthsource* 2008 May; 12(5): 3.

Safir, Michael H., et al. *Overcoming Urinary Incontinence: A Woman's Guide to Treatment.* Addicus Books, 2008.

URINARY TRACT INFECTION (UTI)

During your lifetime, you have at least a 50 percent chance of experiencing a urinary tract infection (UTI), a condition that typically starts in the bladder but may spread to the kidneys. In fact, you may be like many women who can expect to deal with this infection more than once in a lifetime. Fortunately, urinary tract infections are rarely dangerous and are easily treated and prevented.

The urinary system is composed of the bladder, urethra, kidneys, and ureters, all of which have a role in removing waste from your body. The kidneys filter waste from your blood, and tubes called ureters transport urine from your kidneys to your bladder, where it is stored until it leaves your body through the urethra. Although all of these components can become infected, most urinary tract infections are limited to the bladder and urethra.

Symptoms of a UTI depend on the type of infection. Cystitis is an infection or inflammation of the bladder that typically causes lower abdominal discomfort, frequent and painful urination, strong-smelling urine, and pelvic pressure. Urethritis is an infection or inflammation of the urethra that causes burning with urination. If your infection spreads past the urethra and bladder and into the kidneys, this can be a much more serious condition (called acute pyelonephritis) and often has symptoms that include high fever, shaking chills, nausea or vomiting, and upper back and flank pain.

CAUSES AND RISK FACTORS

Women are at greater risk for developing urinary tract infections mainly because they have a shorter urethra than men have, which significantly reduces the distance bacteria must travel to reach the bladder. Other risk factors for urinary tract infections include use of a diaphragm and/or spermicidal products, sexual activity (the risk increases as the amount of sexual activity increases), menopause (loss of estrogen makes the urethra and bladder more fragile), diabetes or other chronic illness, medications that lower immunity (e.g., cortisone, chemotherapy), and use of catheters.

The normal course of a urinary tract infection is for the bacteria to enter the urinary tract through the urethra, travel to the bladder, and multiply. Infection may occur when bacteria commonly found in the digestive system, *Escherichia coli,* get transported to the urethra from the anus when wiping incorrectly (from back to front toward the urethra) after a bowel movement. In cases of urethritis, herpes simplex virus, chlamydia, and other sexually transmitted diseases are also possible causes.

DIAGNOSIS

If you suspect you have a urinary tract infection, contact your doctor as soon as possible. He or she may ask you to bring in a urine sample or to provide one in the office, which can be analyzed (urinalysis and possibly a urine culture) for the presence of bacteria. Diagnosis can be made based on symptoms and the lab report.

PREVENTION AND TREATMENT

To reduce your risk of urinary tract infections, consider these tips:

- **Drink lots of liquids, especially water.** Unsweetened cranberry juice may provide some protection, as it contains potent infection-fighting phytonutrients. Avoid cranberry juice, however, if you are taking the blood-thinning drug warfarin.

- **Wipe from front to back after using the bathroom.** This helps prevent the spread of bacteria from the anal region to the vagina and urethra.

- **Urinate promptly when the urge arises.** If you avoid urinating, you increase the chance of an infection developing in your bladder.

- **Empty your bladder as soon as possible after sexual intercourse.** It is also recommended that you drink a full glass of water to help eliminate bacteria from your body.

- **Do not use irritating feminine products.** Douches, feminine deodorant sprays and powders, and other products designed to cover up vaginal odors can irritate the urethra and other sensitive tissues. A nonirritating soap and water should be sufficient.

The treatment most often prescribed for a UTI for women who are in good health and who have typical symptoms is antibiotics. Your doctor will choose an antibiotic based on your health and the type of bacteria found in your urine. The antibiotics most often recommended for simple UTIs are amoxicillin, nitrofurantoin, trimethoprim, and a combination of trimethoprim and sulfamethoxazole. Symptoms usually resolve within a few days of treatment, but you should take the full course of medication that your doctor prescribed to make sure the infection is completely eliminated.

If you are among the group of women who has recurrent UTIs, your doctor may recommend that you take a longer course of antibiotics. If your infection is severe, treatment with intravenous antibiotics in a hospital may be necessary.

SELF-HELP AND COMPLEMENTARY CARE
Several natural remedies may help prevent and treat a urinary tract infection.

- Unsweetened cranberry or blueberry juice contains potent antioxidants that can prevent and fight infection. Drink up to 16 ounces daily. It is important that the juice be *unsweetened,* as sugar promotes infection.

- Uva ursi is an herb that has been used successfully for urinary tract infections. Drink three to four cups of tea daily, made from 2 teaspoons of dried herb per 8 ounces of hot water. You can also use the tincture (1 to 2 teaspoons in warm water daily).

- Goldenseal root has a long history as an antimicrobial agent. Drink three to four cups of the tea daily made from 1 teaspoon of dried herb per 8 ounces of hot water. You can also take capsules (1,000 mg daily) or tincture (1 to 2 teaspoons in warm water daily).

READ MORE ABOUT IT

Jepson RG, Craig JC. A systematic review of the evidence for cranberries and blueberries in UTI prevention. *Mol Nutr Food Res* 2007 Jun; 51(6): 738–45.

Kilmartin, Angela. *The Patient's Encyclopedia of Urinary Tract Infection, Sexual Cystitis, and Interstitial Cystitis.* New Century Press, 2004.

Moore, Michael. *Herbs for the Urinary Tract.* McGraw-Hill, 1999.

VAGINAL ATROPHY

When estrogen production declines, especially after menopause, the walls of the vagina can become thin and inflamed. This condition, called vaginal atrophy or atrophic vaginitis, affects more than half of menopausal women. Very few seek treatment, however, often out of embarrassment, even though the condition makes intercourse painful and may even lead to urinary tract infections or urinary incontinence (see "Urinary Tract Infection" and "Urinary Incontinence").

Not every woman who has vaginal atrophy experiences symptoms that are troublesome, but if the condition becomes more advanced, some of the symptoms you may experience include vaginal dryness and burning, a watery vaginal discharge, burning and/or urgency with urination, a tendency to get frequent urinary tract infections, light bleeding after intercourse, and painful intercourse. Vaginal atrophy can also cause your vaginal canal to become shorter and narrower.

CAUSES AND RISK FACTORS

You increase your chances of getting vaginal atrophy if you smoke, because smoking interferes with blood circulation and deprives your tissues of oxygen; smoking also reduces the effects of natural estrogens and makes you less responsive to oral estrogen therapy. Surgical removal of your ovaries lowers the level of testosterone, which may lead to vaginal atrophy.

Another risk factor for vaginal atrophy is having never given birth vaginally.

Vaginal atrophy is caused by a significant decline in estrogen levels, which makes your vaginal tissues drier, less elastic, thinner, and more fragile. The most common cause of reduced estrogen levels is menopause. That's not to say that premenopausal women do not develop vaginal atrophy. In fact, women who are breast-feeding, have had pelvic radiation for cancer, have received chemotherapy, or have had both ovaries removed may also experience vaginal atrophy.

DIAGNOSIS
Your doctor will ask about your symptoms and do a complete pelvic examination, during which he or she will look for signs of vaginal atrophy, prolapse, and any other abnormalities. He or she may order a blood test to assess your hormone status and take a sample of cells from your vagina to check for infection.

PREVENTION AND TREATMENT
The best way to prevent vaginal atrophy is to engage in sexual intercourse on a regular basis. Sexual activity enhances blood flow and helps keep vaginal tissues healthy.

If you are not experiencing any vaginal discomfort, you probably don't need treatment. However, if you have discomfort such as vaginal dryness, irritation, pain with intercourse, urinary urgency, or urinary frequency, then some treatments are available for you. The most effective treatment is application of a topical (cream) estrogen to the vaginal area. Another option is local estrogen therapy, which comes in the form of slow-releasing vaginal suppositories or rings that stay in place for up to three months. Although you may absorb some estrogen into your bloodstream when you first start local estrogen therapy, the amount you continue to absorb will decline. This form of estrogen therapy does not usually affect the uterine lining, as seen with systemic (pill, gel, patch) estrogen therapy.

If your vaginal atrophy is accompanied by hot flashes, sleep problems, or night sweats, systemic estrogen therapy (preferably natural estrogen) may be a better choice for you. If you still have your uterus, you need to take progestin (natural progesterone preferred) as well to reduce your risk of endometrial cancer and breast cancer. With either form of estrogen therapy, you should notice some improvement within a few weeks.

SELF-HELP AND COMPLEMENTARY CARE
Several over-the-counter products are available that can relieve vaginal dryness and irritation. Products such as K-Y, Silk-E, and Replens can be used regularly to restore some moisture to your vaginal area. Water-based lubricants, such as Astroglide, can reduce discomfort during sex. Do not use petroleum-based products if you also use condoms, as the petroleum can break down latex and make the condoms ineffective.

READ MORE ABOUT IT
Cicinelli E. Intravaginal oestrogen and progestin administration: advantages and disadvantages. *Bes Pract Res Clin Obstet Gynaecol* 2008 Apr; 22(2): 391–405.

North American Menopause Society. The role of local vaginal estrogen for treatment of vaginal atrophy in postmenopausal women: 2007 position statement of The North American Menopause Society. *Menopause* 2007 May–Jun; 14(3 pt 1): 355–69.

VAGINAL YEAST INFECTION

A vaginal yeast infection is an irritation of the vagina and the surrounding area (vulva) associated with an overgrowth of a fungus or yeast. About 75 percent of women have a yeast infection at some point in their lives, and nearly half of all women have two or more infections during their lifetime.

If you have ever had a vaginal yeast infection, you know what we mean when we say the main symptom is an extreme itchiness in and around the vagina that can completely disrupt your life. You can't sit still; you can't go out in public; you may miss days at work or school. Other symptoms include burning and swelling of the vagina and vulva, pain when urinating, pain or discomfort during sex, and a thick, odorless, cottage-cheese-like discharge from the vagina. You may have one or more of these symptoms, and they can be mild to severe.

CAUSES AND RISK FACTORS

Every time Claudia took a course of antibiotics for an infection, she ended up with a yeast infection soon after she finished her medication. After the third yeast infection episode, she went online and did some research. It didn't take her long to learn that taking antibiotics was destroying the good bacteria and other healthy flora in her body and that she was opening herself up for a yeast infection whenever she took antibiotics.

Taking antibiotics is not the only risk factor for vaginal yeast infections. Others include uncontrolled diabetes (the presence of sugar supports yeast growth), pregnancy, using contraceptives high in estrogen, thyroid or endocrine disorders, and use of corticosteroid therapy.

The organism that causes vaginal yeast infections is *Candida albicans*. This fungus takes hold when you have a weakened immune system, as occurs when taking antibiotics. Other factors that can contribute to a weakened system include stress, poor nutrition (especially eating sugary foods), lack of sleep, and chronic illness.

DIAGNOSIS

Candidiasis is not hard to diagnose: the signs of swelling and telltale, odorous vaginal discharge are usually very revealing, and your doctor can quickly verify the presence of yeast by taking a swab sample from your vagina and looking at it under a microscope or sending it to a lab for analysis.

PREVENTION AND TREATMENT

You can help prevent yeast infections by following some simple guidelines:

- Do not use douches or scented hygiene products (e.g., bubble bath, sprays, tampons, pads, powders).

- Change your tampon or pad often during your period.

- Wear cotton underwear and pantyhose with a cotton crotch.

- Change out of wet swimsuits and clothes as soon as possible.

- After using the toilet, always wipe from front to back.

- Avoid sugary foods, alcohol, and processed foods.

Yeast infections can be eliminated with antifungal medications that can be purchased over the counter (OTC) or by prescription in the form of creams, tablets, ointments, or suppositories that are inserted into the vagina. The OTC medications include butoconazole, clotrimazole, miconazole, nystatin, tioconazole, and terconazole. A cautionary word about using OTC medications is that you don't want to use them if you don't really have a yeast infection, because it can increase your risk of getting a difficult-to-treat infection in the future. You should verify your self-diagnosis with your doctor before starting treatment if it is practical to do so. As an alternative to OTC medications, your doctor can prescribe a single dose of oral fluconazole.

SELF-HELP AND COMPLEMENTARY CARE
Several studies and numerous anecdotal reports tell of the benefits of taking probiotics (beneficial bacteria) to help prevent and treat vaginal yeast infections and other forms of vaginitis. The beneficial bacteria found to be helpful in fighting vaginal yeast infections include *Lactobacillus acidophilus, L. delbrueckii, L. plantarum, L. rhamnosus,* and *L. fermentum.* Look for products that contain at least two of these species of bacteria. If you have an active infection, a recommended dose, according to John T. Taylor, author of *The Wonder of Probiotics,* is 16.5 billion CFUs (colony-forming units, a standard measurement for probiotics) per meal for five days, then 11 billion CFUs per meal for five more days, then 5.5 billion CFUs per meal until your symptoms are under control. If you want to help prevent yeast infections in the future, you can stay on a maintenance dose of 2 billion CFUs daily, preferably with your morning meal.

READ MORE ABOUT IT
Burton, G. *The Candida Control Cookbook: What You Should Know and What You Should Eat to Manage Yeast Infections.* 3rd ed. Aslan Publishing, 2002.

Falagas ME et al. Probiotics for prevention of recurrent vulvovaginal candidiasis: a review. *J Antimicrob Chemother* 2006 Aug; 58(2): 266–72.

Martin, Jeanne Marie, and Zoltan P. Rona. *Complete Candida Yeast Guidebook: Everything You Need to Know About Prevention, Treatment, and Diet.* 2nd ed. Three Rivers Press, 2000.

Vaginitis. *See* "Bacterial Vaginosis," "Trichomoniasis," "Vaginal Atrophy," "Vaginal Yeast Infection."

Q&A

Having sexual intercourse regularly (once or twice a week) is said to help prevent vaginal atrophy, but what about masturbation? Is that helpful too?

Although there is little research to support this statement, masturbation may help maintain vaginal secretions and elasticity. For women who do not have a sexual partner but who want to avoid vaginal atrophy, masturbation is an option.

This may sound like a strange question, but how do I choose a tampon? There are so many different absorbency ratings, applicators, and questions about deodorant versus non-deodorant.

First, you should choose a tampon that is only as absorbent as you need. To determine which absorbency rating is best for you, note how long it takes a tampon to become saturated. If it is not saturated after four to six hours, switch to one that's less absorbent. Manufacturers have several "grades" of absorbency: junior, regular, super, and super plus. An entire menstrual period usually produces 4 to 12 teaspoons of fluid, which weighs about 20 to 60 grams (1 teaspoon is about 5 grams). The least absorbent tampons can handle less than 6 grams; regular tampons can absorb about 6 to 9 grams, super from 9 to 12 grams, and super plus from 12 to 15 grams. During any given menstrual period, you will likely need several different types of tampons, each with a different absorbency rating, as your flow rate will change.

Second, do not use scented, deodorant tampons. Chemically treated tampons do not belong in the vagina, as they may cause irritation and discomfort. You should also use tampons only when you have your period and only if you have not had toxic shock syndrome in the past.

Finally, some tampon applicators have rounded tips (typically plastic applicators), while others do not (usually paper/cardboard applicators); some have no applicators. While many women find the rounded tips more comfortable, others find either or no applicator acceptable. This is a personal choice.

How accurate are Pap smears? I'm thrilled that the results of my latest test were negative, but what if they're wrong?

You're right to question the reliability of Pap smear results, as there are conflicting reports on their accuracy. On one hand, there are generally accepted figures that negative results are correct 99.4 percent of the time, and that positive results are right 80 percent of the time. On the other hand, some research indicates that negative results are correct only 69 percent of the time and that a positive finding is correct around 58 percent of the time.

About two-thirds of false negative results (which means the report says you don't have cervical disease but you do) are caused by poor collection and/or handling or evaluation of the sample. Sampling errors can occur when the clinician takes the sample and transfers it to a slide, or the lab may not detect abnormal cells that are there.

A newer technology can reduce the error margin. It is called ThinPrep, and rather than smear the sample on a slide, the clinician swirls the sample in a container that contains a special solution. This action reduces the amount of cells that can be lost when the swab used to collect the sample is discarded, and it also cuts down on residual matter such as blood and mucus that might "contaminate" the sample. In the lab, the cells are collected and transferred to a microscope slide, and the slide sample tends to be much clearer than the traditional method. ThinPrep is more costly than the traditional collection method, and it is not always covered by insurance. Some clinicians use it as a follow-up test when their patients get a positive result on their first test.

If you are concerned, you can always ask for a second Pap test. However, you should know that the industry-accepted way to reduce errors is to simply have an annual Pap test. The proportion of false negatives declines to less than 1 percent for women who have three consecutive annual Pap smears. Two-thirds of women who develop cervical cancer did not have a Pap test in five years, or ever.

I have very lumpy breasts and they are often tender. I've been told I have fibrocystic breasts. Is there anything I can do in my diet to help reduce the discomfort and the lumps?

Although hormones are the main culprits in fibrocystic breast changes, many women find that making some dietary modifications can be very helpful in relieving symptoms and reducing lumpiness. Eliminating caffeine, foods containing saturated fats, and salt have lead to significant improvement for many women, as has eating many plant-based, high-fiber foods. The addition of cold-water fatty fish such as salmon, mackerel, and sardines is also said to be helpful, as they contain high amounts of omega-3 fatty acids, which help reduce inflammation.

You may also want to take supplements of vitamin E (500 to 600 IU daily), which has been shown to reduce pain and tenderness as well as the size of breast lumps. Several studies have found that evening primrose oil, a source of the essential fatty acid linoleic acid and its derivative, gamma-linolenic acid, provides symptom relief. A typical dose is 1,500 mg twice daily.

Why are so many doctors down on douching? Isn't it good for getting rid of vaginal odors?

Routine bathing or showering with mild soap and water is more than adequate to keep your genital area clean. The vagina is self-cleaning, so you don't need to introduce anything into it to keep it clean. Most vaginal odor is caused by yeast or bacterial vaginosis, and douching actually can make these conditions worse by pushing these infections higher into the body. Women who douche once or twice a week also have about a fourfold increased risk of developing pelvic inflammatory disease. We also want to emphasize that douching is not a form of birth control, nor can it prevent sexually transmitted diseases.

I am thirty-eight years old and have four children. Recently I've noticed some urine leakage, especially whenever I laugh hard or sneeze or when I'm jogging, which I took up to help me lose weight. Now I'm afraid to go out because I don't want to embarrass myself. I don't want to wear pads all the time. What can I do?

It appears that your four pregnancies and childbirth experiences have left your pelvic floor muscles less than taut. This is entirely natural, but that doesn't mean you can't do something about it, and it likely won't involve the use of drugs or an invasive procedure. All you may need is Kegel exercises.

Kegel exercises, which are discussed in part II, are simple yet effective exercises you can do just about anywhere, at any time, and no one will know you're doing them. Once you learn the technique, which we explain but you can read about in a variety of places both online and in print, you can do the exercises several times a day for just a few minutes at a time. You will probably need to use pads for a short time if you are worried about leakage, but after a few months of daily exercise, you could very likely be pad-free and worry-free.

I've had severe premenstrual symptoms for months, and I've been trying to treat them myself. A friend told me I might have PMDD. What is PMDD and can I get help?

Approximately 3 to 8 percent of women have supersized PMS, a condition known as premenstrual dysphoric disorder, or PMDD. The symptoms of PMDD are the same as PMS symptoms, but women with PMDD experience five or more symptoms and they are more severe. According to the American Psychiatric Association, a diagnosis of PMDD requires that the symptoms be severe enough to disrupt a woman's daily activities, and the most critical symptoms are those associated with mood—severe mood swings, anxiety, depression, loss of interest in daily life, crying spells, severe sleep difficulties, feelings of hopelessness and helplessness, and more. Women who have a history of depression are at greater risk for PMDD.

No one should have to suffer with PMDD. Treatment includes use of the antidepressant medications called selective serotonin reuptake inhibitors (SSRIs), and a newly FDA-approved type of birth control pills that contain drospirenone (a progestin) along with ethinyl estradiol are effective in relieving the emotional and physical symptoms of PMDD.

What's the difference between synthetic and natural progesterone?

Natural progesterone—that is, the hormone produced naturally by the body—is referred to as progesterone. The synthetic hormone is called progestin, which you may recognize by the name medroxyprogesterone, commonly prescribed as Provera. The chemical structure of medroxyprogesterone is close to but not exactly like that of progesterone, and that small modification makes a big difference when it comes to impact on the body. In fact, medroxyprogesterone can actually reduce your blood level of progesterone. Some women who take medroxyprogesterone to treat PMS symptoms experience fluid retention, mood swings, and headache. Women who take natural progesterone, however, report relief from mood swings, migraine, and fluid retention.

The natural progesterone that is available as a hormone supplement is made from yams and soybeans, based on a process discovered by a chemistry professor named Russell Marker back in the 1930s. The natural micronized (made into minute particles readily used by the body) progesterone available today is an exact chemical duplicate of the progesterone produced by your body.

Someone told me that natural progesterone can help my endometriosis. Does it really work?

Some women find that their endometriosis symptoms are greatly reduced when they use natural progesterone cream. The reason is that while estrogen stimulates endometriosis, progesterone inhibits it. You want to use natural progesterone, not progestins (e.g., medroxyprogesterone), because you want to mimic the body's natural response to the progesterone. Progestins cause side effects and do not mimic the natural process.

One clue to progesterone's ability to relieve endometriosis comes from pregnancy: when a woman who has endometriosis gets pregnant, her symptoms usually disappear, only to return after pregnancy. This suggests that the very high progesterone levels that occur during pregnancy are key in inhibiting the disease. Therefore, for women with endometriosis, progesterone (as a cream) is often recommended from days eight to twenty-six, just before menstruation begins. Typically, high doses are needed to control pain, around 60 to 80mg daily, although you should consult with your health care provider to determine the best dose for you. Women who use progesterone cream for endometriosis find that they need to keep using the hormone; if they stop, after several months the supply of progesterone in their body is depleted and the disease flares up again.

I hear a lot about endometrial (uterine) cancer, ovarian cancer, and cervical cancer, but what about vaginal cancer? Is there such a thing?

Primary vaginal cancer—cancer that originates in the vagina—is rare, affecting less than 2,500 women in the United States per year. Women most likely to get vaginal cancer are those whose mothers took diethylstilbestrol (DES) when they were pregnant. DES was prescribed in the 1950s to prevent miscarriages and had this unfortunate and unknown side effect. Vaginal cancer is also more common in women sixty and older and among women who have had human papillomavirus (HPV) infection. Some women who have vaginal cancer got it because it metastasized from another location in the body.

How effective is cranberry juice for preventing or treating urinary tract infections? Should I make cranberry juice part of my diet?

Drink up! Numerous studies have shown that both cranberry and blueberry juice are helpful in preventing and treating urinary tract infections. At one time experts thought that the vitamin C in cranberries and their acidic nature were the reasons why this fruit was so effective against urinary tract infections. Now researchers have determined that it is because of compounds called condensed tannins (more specifically, proanthocyanidins) that are found in cranberries, blueberries, and several other fruit species. These tannins prevent the disease-causing organisms called P-fimbriated *Escherichia coli* from attaching to the walls of the urinary tract.

Not everyone agrees on the amount of cranberry and/or blueberry juice you need to consume to prevent or treat urinary tract infections, but generally two to three 8--ounce glasses of unsweetened juice are suggested. Because many women don't want the calories that go along with the juice, there is an alternative: concentrated cranberry extract found in supplements. Studies show that taking 200 mg of concentrated cranberry extract (standardized at 30 percent phenolics) twice a day protects against urinary tract infections. Of course, you can mix it up and drink a glass of juice and take one supplement as an alternative. Concentrated blueberry extracts are also available; look for those standardized at 2.5 percent anthocyanins. The usual dose is one to three 500 mg capsules daily.

I have had genital herpes for five years and I just found out I'm pregnant. I'm worried about my baby getting infected,

*but I really don't want to have a C-section. What are the
chances that my baby will get herpes?*

First of all, your doctor needs to know that you have
herpes, if you haven't revealed it already. He or she will
know how to handle the situation and can advise you
throughout your pregnancy about how to take care of
yourself and your options when it comes time to deliver.

Here are some facts that can help you feel better about
your situation. An estimated 20 to 25 percent of pregnant women have genital herpes, yet less than 0.1 percent of babies get the disease from their mothers. The
risk of passing the infection to your infant is high if you
have an active, symptomatic outbreak of herpes at the
time of delivery. There is also a small risk of transmitting the disease if the virus reactivates without causing
any symptoms.

Nature has a way of taking care of her own, however, and
babies of mothers who have long-standing herpes infections are naturally protected against the virus because
herpes antibodies cross the placenta from the mother
to the fetus. These antibodies help protect the baby
from getting the infection during birth, and they are the
main reason why mothers who have recurrent genital
herpes episodes rarely transmit the disease to their babies during delivery. If your baby is born prematurely,
he or she may be at slightly greater risk because the
transfer of antibodies from you to your child begins at
about twenty-eight weeks of pregnancy and continues
until birth; premature babies do not get the benefit of all
the antibodies.

You are fortunate because you've had herpes for some
time (I bet you didn't think there was any advantage to
having herpes at all!) and so you will be producing an-

tibodies and passing them along to your child at around twenty-eight weeks. In contrast, mothers who acquire genital herpes during the last trimester of pregnancy often don't have the time to make enough antibodies, and those who get the disease during the last few weeks of pregnancy are at the highest risk of transmitting the virus to their infants.

Hot flashes are my biggest complaint in menopause, and I don't want to take hormones. What is the best herbal treatment for hot flashes?

We investigated what the experts have to say, and there are about a dozen herbs that many naturopaths and herbalists find to be helpful. We've narrowed it down to four that seem to make everyone's list.

- **Dong quai** is reportedly good not only for hot flashes but for mood swings as well. It appears that dong quai helps hot flashes because it helps to stabilize the blood vessels. A recommended dose is one 500 mg tablet or capsule twice daily, or ½ teaspoon of tincture twice daily. Dong quai works best for women who have intermittent hot flashes rather than women who are hot much of the time.

- **Chasteberry** (vitex) helps reduce estrogen levels and increases both progesterone and the brain chemical dopamine. It is a slow-acting herb, as it takes about two to three months of use before you will notice improvement. A suggested dose is 300 to 600 mg in tablet or capsule form daily, or ½ teaspoon of tincture twice daily.

- **Black cohosh** is one herb that has held up under scientific scrutiny and is effective not only for hot flashes but for vaginal atrophy and depression also. A suggested dose is 10 to 15 drops of extract once or twice daily or one 250 mg tablet or capsule two to four times daily, for several months.

- **Licorice** is believed to reduce estrogen levels while boosting progesterone. The major component of licorice, glycyrrhizin, regulates estrogen metabolism. Licorice is a powerful drug and should not be used for more than four to six weeks at a time. The suggested dose for hot flashes is one 500 or 1,000 mg tablet or capsule daily; ½ to 1 teaspoon of tincture, twice daily; or one to two cups of licorice tea daily.

PART II

Tests, Procedures, Surgeries, and Devices

ABORTION

The common definition of *abortion* is the intentional or elected termination of a pregnancy, although technically the term includes unintentional loss of the fetus as well, as when a miscarriage occurs. (In this entry we discuss intentional termination only; see "Miscarriage" in Part I.) An intentional abortion is a controversial issue that brings up many moral and legal arguments both for and against the procedures that result in the termination of a pregnancy.

In the United States, approximately one-third of women have had an abortion by the time they are 45 years old. Until recently, those abortions, when performed by medical professionals, were accomplished by a medical procedure. Today, there is a second approach to abortion, by way of an abortion pill.

More than 1.2 million abortions are performed in the United States every year. If you are considering an abortion, bear in mind that the earlier it is performed—and when it is done by a knowledgeable medical professional—the safer it is.

HOW TO PREPARE

Before you undergo abortion by any method, you should discuss your options with a trusted medical professional and other important people in your life to make sure you understand your choices and the consequences. Your doctor will evaluate your medical history, order lab tests, and perform a physical examination, which usually includes an ultrasound. If you plan to take a sedative for the procedure, you should arrange to have someone drive you home.

HOW IT IS DONE

There are two types of intentional abortion: abortion by pill (medication) and abortion by procedure. The abortion pill is mifepristone, or RU-486, and can be taken up to sixty-three days after the first day of your last period. It is effective 97 percent of the time. Antibiotics are prescribed along with the abortion pill to help prevent any risk of infection. If mifepristone does not successfully end the pregnancy, then an *aspiration abortion* (see below) will need to be performed.

If you choose abortion by a medical procedure, there are two main approaches: aspiration and D&E (dilation and evacuation). Aspiration, also called vacuum aspiration, makes up more than 90 percent of the abortions performed in the United States. An aspiration procedure takes about five to ten minutes, although more time may be needed to prepare your cervix. Recovery is about one hour. Generally, the procedure is as follows:

- Your health care provider examines your uterus and gives you medication for pain and possibly a sedative. Antibiotics are also given to prevent infection.

- A speculum is inserted into your vagina and a numbing medication is injected near your cervix.

- Your cervix may be stretched with dilators and a tube is inserted through the cervix into the uterus.

- The clinician uses a suction device to gently empty your uterus.

- An instrument called a curette (used to perform a D&C) may be used to remove any tissue that may have remained behind.

Dilation and evacuation is usually performed later than 16 weeks after a woman's last period. Less than 10 percent of all abortions in the United States are D&Es. The procedure takes between ten and twenty minutes, although it may take additional time to prepare the cervix. A D&E procedure is similar to aspiration abortion, but once your cervix has been stretched, the health care provider will use both a suction device and instruments to perform the procedure. If the D&E is being done late in the second trimester, your clinician may give you an injection in your abdomen before proceeding to ensure the demise of the fetus. Recovery time is about one hour.

RISKS/SIDE EFFECTS
After an abortion procedure, it is common to experience some heavy bleeding for a few days and spotting for up to six weeks. You may also have some cramping and pass clots about the size of a quarter. If, however, you experience fever, vomiting for more than four to six hours, very heavy bleeding, or passing of very large clots, seek medical assistance immediately.

READ MORE ABOUT IT
Bachiochi, Erika. *The Cost of Choice: Women Evaluate the Impact of Abortion.* Encounter Books, 2004.

Lipp A. A review of developments in medical termination of pregnancy. *J Clin Nurs* 2008 Jun; 17(11): 1411–18.

AMNIOCENTESIS

Some pregnant women undergo amniocentesis, a diagnostic test typically used to help prospective parents determine if specific genetic or inherited disorders may be present in their baby. It is usually done when women are between sixteen and twenty weeks pregnant.

HOW TO PREPARE
There is no preparation needed for amniocentesis. However, you should talk to your health care provider about any questions or concerns you have about the procedure.

HOW IT IS DONE
Amniocentesis involves inserting a needle into the amniotic sac so that fluid can be safely removed for analysis. The test is usually performed between fourteen and twenty weeks, although some facilities may do the procedure as early as eleven weeks if necessary. Amniocentesis can also be done late in the third trimester if your membranes have ruptured prematurely or to detect the severity of fetal anemia in infants that have Rh disease. It can also be performed soon before delivery to check your infant's lung function.

Your health care provider will use ultrasound to determine the position of the fetus and the placenta and to guide placement of the needle. Although actual collection of the fluid takes about five minutes, the entire procedure lasts about forty-five minutes because it takes time to set up the procedure. The amniotic fluid sample, which contains cells shed by the fetus, is analyzed in a lab.

BENEFITS
Amniocentesis allows prospective parents to determine whether their child may be born with an inherited or genetic condition, such as spina bifida, Down syndrome, sickle cell disease, hemophilia, or cystic fibrosis. Overall, amniocentesis can detect several hundred different genetic disorders and nearly all chromosomal disorders. This test has an accuracy rate of 98 to 99 percent, although it cannot measure the severity of the birth defects. To help determine severity, your health care provider may order advanced ultrasound tests or an alpha-fetoprotein test. Amniocentesis cannot detect birth defects caused by your exposure to X-rays, rubella, drugs, or other harmful substances.

RISKS/SIDE EFFECTS
According to the Mayo Clinic, amniocentesis is performed approximately 200,000 times a year. The main risk is miscarriage, which ranges from 1 in 400 to 1 in 200, and it occurs because of infection, the water breaking prematurely, or labor being induced too early. In extremely rare cases, the needle touches the baby, but the use of ultrasound helps prevent this from happening.

Side effects from the procedure may include a sharp pain when the needle enters the skin and again when it enters the uterus. After the procedure, you may experience cramping, minor irritation around the puncture site, and leakage of fluid.

READ MORE ABOUT IT
ICON Health Publications. *Amniocentesis: A Medical Dictionary, Bibliography, and Annotated Research Guide to Internet References.* ICON Health Publications, 2003.

Zalud I, Janas S. Risks of third-trimester amniocentesis. *J Reprod Med* 2008 Jan; 53(1): 45–48.

ARTIFICIAL INSEMINATION

Artificial insemination is a general term that includes various techniques used to place sperm into the female genital tract. Insemination may be intravaginal, intracervical, intrauterine, intrafallopian, and intraperitoneal (in which sperm are placed inside the pelvis near the mouth of the fallopian tubes and ovaries). The most commonly used techniques are intrauterine, intracervical, and intravaginal insemination. Intrauterine insemination has a higher success rate than the other techniques because the sperm are placed near the fallopian tubes.

Artificial insemination is used for a variety of circumstances, the most common of which is the inability of the male to ejaculate inside the woman's vagina. Causes for this failure may include diabetes, multiple sclerosis, retrograde ejaculation (when sperm travels backward into the bladder instead of out through the urethra), or spinal cord injury. Men who have a mildly low sperm count, antisperm antibodies, or poor-quality sperm also may participate in artificial insemination. Couples with unexplained infertility, women with mild endometriosis, and women who have poor cervical mucus also are candidates for artificial insemination.

HOW TO PREPARE
To improve your chance of becoming pregnant, your doctor will likely prescribe a fertility drug before you undergo artifi-

cial insemination. You should take this drug near the beginning of your menstrual cycle.

HOW IT IS DONE

For artificial insemination to have a chance to be successful, you need to be inseminated while you are ovulating. To find out if you are ovulating, you can use an ovulation detection kit or your doctor may perform an ultrasound. Once you are ovulating, your partner will provide a sperm sample, which will be processed so that only the most viable sperm will be used. These sperm are mixed with a small amount of fluid, and the mixture is put directly into your uterus through your cervix using a catheter. Two weeks later you can take a pregnancy test to see if insemination has been successful.

Although the insemination takes less than one hour, you may have to take fertility drugs for a week or more before you ovulate. Most women need to undergo three to six cycles of artificial insemination before they get pregnant.

BENEFITS

For couples dealing with infertility, artificial insemination is often the first step because it is less invasive and less expensive than other options, including in vitro fertilization (IVF; see "In Vitro Fertilization"). Research shows that couples who have unexplained fertility problems get better results with artificial insemination than by using fertility drugs alone.

RISKS/SIDE EFFECTS

The timing of artificial insemination is crucial: it requires that both you and your partner must be ready to go to your doctor's office when you are ovulating, and your partner must be able to supply a sperm sample on demand at your doctor's office. If you cannot coordinate these factors, then you will have to repeat the cycle again the following month.

READ MORE ABOUT IT

Custers IM et al. Intrauterine insemination: how many cycles should we perform? *Hum Reprod* 2008 Apr; 23(4): 885–88.

Streda R et al. Ovulation induction increases pregnancy rate during intrauterine insemination compared with natural cycles. *Ceska Gynekol* 2007 Dec; 72(6): 397–402.

BIOPSY

A biopsy is the removal of a small amount of tissue from a living person for evaluation and diagnosis. It is the primary diagnostic technique used to evaluate tumors for the presence of cancerous cells. There are basically two types of biopsy—surgical biopsy, of which there are various subtypes, including excisional, punch, cervical, and endometrial; and needle, which does not require an incision.

HOW TO PREPARE
Your health care provider will tell you how you should prepare for your biopsy. Generally, one week before the procedure patients are asked to stop taking any medications that may make you bleed, such as aspirin, warfarin (Coumadin), and nonsteroidal anti-inflammatory drugs (NSAIDs). Tell your doctor about any herbs and other supplements you may be taking. You will be asked to abstain from food for a certain length of time before the procedure, and you may be given antibiotics to ward off any possible infection.

HOW IT IS DONE
Here is a rundown of some types of biopsies and how they are done.

- **Breast biopsy.** The term "breast biopsy" is a general one because there are many different types of breast lumps and tumors, and thus your health care provider will choose the best biopsy method to fit the circumstances. If a breast lump is filled with fluid, for example, the liquid can be extracted using a needle (see "Fine-Needle Aspiration"). If the lump is solid, the clinician will work a needle in and out several times to gather cells for analysis. Deep lumps may require excisional biopsy. Other biopsy techniques, including stereotactic biopsy and wire-localization biopsy, may also be used.

- **Cervical biopsy.** This biopsy is usually an office procedure and does not require any anesthesia. You may experience a mild cramp or two when the sample is taken.

- **Core needle biopsy.** Also called a core biopsy, it is done by inserting a small hollow needle through the skin and into the area to be investigated. The needle may have a cutting tip or there may be a spring-loaded gun to help remove the sample. Core biopsy is usually done under the guidance of CT imaging, ultrasound, or mammography. You may experience slight pressure, but there is generally no significant pain involved. A local anesthetic will be given to numb the insertion site.

- **Endoscopic biopsy.** This is a very common type of biopsy that is done through an endoscope (a fiber-optic cable that allows a clinician to view inside the body). The scope is inserted into the body along with sampling instruments. Endoscopic biopsy can be performed of the urinary bladder (cystoscopy), abdominal cavity (laparoscopy), and several other areas. The clinician can visualize the abnormality and pinch off tissue samples with forceps attached to the cable that is inside the endoscope. You will be given a sedative and/or anesthetic, depending on the type of endoscopic biopsy you undergo.

- **Excisional biopsy.** Removal of an entire growth for evaluation. It is usually done under general anesthesia.

- **Fine-needle aspiration.** A long, thin needle is inserted into the suspicious area and a syringe is used to withdraw the fluid and cells. Clinicians often use X-rays to help guide the needle to the appropriate area. You will get a local anesthetic to numb the insertion site.

- **Punch biopsy.** Removal of a small wedge of tissue using a special device that punches rather than cuts. It is sometimes used to diagnose possible cancer of the cervix.

After the procedure, do not drive for at least one day. Depending on the site of the biopsy, you should not fly the same day as the procedure. Results of your biopsy may take several days to several weeks.

BENEFITS
The results of a biopsy can tell you and your doctor whether the cells are cancerous and if they are, the type of cancer that is present. Biopsy results also reveal how aggressive a cancer is, which can be most helpful in deciding on a treatment course.

RISKS/SIDE EFFECTS
Side effects from a biopsy generally range from none to mild. Some people experience slight to moderate pain, which can be controlled with acetaminophen; do not take aspirin or NSAIDs until forty-eight hours after the procedure. If you have had an excisional biopsy, you may experience some irritation at the incision site or the stitches may be itchy. A cone biopsy is an exception, in that you may experience cramping and mild to moderate bleeding for a few weeks after the procedure. You should abstain from sexual intercourse, douching, and the use of tampons for several weeks after the biopsy to allow the area to heal.

READ MORE ABOUT IT
Feoli F et al. Fine needle aspiration cytology of the breast: impact of experience on accuracy, using standardized cytologic criteria. *Acta Cytol* 2008 Mar–Apr; 52(2): 145–51.

Philipotts LE. Percutaneous breast biopsy: emerging techniques and continuing controversies. *Semin Roentgenol* 2007 Oct; 42(4): 218–27.

Birth Control. *See* "Birth Control Pills," "Diaphragm," "Intrauterme Device"; also see "Effectiveness of Birth Control Methods" in Part III.

BIRTH CONTROL PILLS

Birth control pills are the number one choice among women as a means of birth control, or contraception. There are many different brands of the pill, each containing a specific and different amount of synthetic estrogen and/or progestin (synthetic progesterone). Every woman has unique needs when it comes to a hormonal form of birth control, so it can take several tries before you and your physician find the right pill for your needs. You will be choosing from the following main categories of birth control pills:

- **Progestin-only pills.** Also called minipills, they are typically used by breast-feeding women because estrogen reduces their milk production. They are also used by women who cannot take estrogen.

- **Monophasic pills.** Twenty-one of the pills in this pack contain the same amount of estrogen and progestin; the other seven are placebos, and menstruation occurs while you take these seven. Also available is a ninety-one-day pill program in which you take the combination pills for eighty-four days and the placebo for seven days. With this product, you menstruate about once every three months.

- **Multiphasic pills.** Also called biphasic or triphasic, these pills contain varied amounts of hormones and are taken at specific times throughout the program. These pills were developed to help reduce the side effects associated with higher levels of hormones in some oral contraceptives.

- **Continuous-use pills.** This is a type of multiphasic that is taken continuously, with no placebos. If you take this pill, you will not have a period, but you may experience spotting or breakthrough bleeding.

- **Morning-after pill.** This form of emergency birth control prevents women from becoming pregnant after unprotected vaginal intercourse. The morning-after pill can be taken within seventy-two hours of intercourse with a second dose taken twelve hours later. It is reportedly more than eighty percent effective in preventing pregnancy after a single act of unprotected sex. It is not the same as the so-called abortion pill (mifepristone).

HOW TO PREPARE
A health care provider must provide a prescription for the pill for you. He or she should give you a physical examination and review your medical history before choosing the hormone combination for you.

As your doctor can discuss with you, some women should not take the pill. For example, taking the pill places some women at risk for serious health problems. If you are older than thirty-five and smoke, or if you have any of the following conditions, you should not take the pill:

- History of blood clots or a circulatory disorder associated with blood clots

- History of stroke or heart attack

- Unexplained vaginal bleeding

- Pregnancy or suspected pregnancy

- Known or suspected cancer

- Liver or kidney disease

- Moderate to severe hypertension

- Severe migraine

If you are younger than thirty-five and smoke and have hypertension, migraines, gallbladder disease, diabetes, epilepsy, sickle cell disease, or a history of blood clots or heart disease, use of the pill may place you in jeopardy. Talk to your doctor about your choices.

HOW IT PERFORMS

At the beginning of each menstrual cycle, estrogen levels rise, causing the endometrium to thicken in preparation for a fertilized egg. After about fourteen days, the ovaries release an egg (ovulation), after which progesterone levels begin to rise. This hormone also prepares the endometrium for a fertilized egg. If a fertilized egg implants itself in the endometrium, conception occurs; if not, the levels of estrogen and progesterone decline and menstruation begins. The pill stops ovulation by preventing the ovaries from releasing eggs. It also causes the mucus in the cervix to thicken, which makes it difficult for sperm to enter the uterus.

BENEFITS

Oral contraceptives are easy to use, don't require you to interrupt your sexual activity, and don't jeopardize future fertility. Birth control pills also offer a host of benefits beyond preventing pregnancy. Combination pills, for example:

- Reduce the risk of ovarian and endometrial cancer and ovarian cysts

- Decrease menstrual blood loss, pain, and cramping

- Help regulate your menstrual cycles

- Improve acne

- Prevent bone density loss in women older than thirty

- Prevent ectopic pregnancy

- Improve endometriosis

- Improve symptoms of rheumatoid arthritis

- Have a beneficial impact on high-density lipoprotein (HDL) and low-density lipoprotein (LDL) cholesterol levels

- Reduce the risk of benign breast disease and breast cysts

The progestin-only pills also have some benefits, including decreased menstrual blood loss, cramps, and pain, and they can be used by nursing women immediately after delivery.

RISKS/SIDE EFFECTS

Women often experience some minor side effects when they start taking the pill as their body adjusts to the hormonal changes the pill causes. Those who take the progestin-only pills may experience irregular bleeding, heavy bleeding, abdominal pain, headache, and amenorrhea. Women who choose the combination pills may have headache, irregular bleeding, weight gain or weight loss, breast tenderness, an increase in breast size, nausea, and vomiting. With both types of pills, side effects typically disappear after two to three months.

READ MORE ABOUT IT

Kiley J, Hammond C. Combined oral contraceptives: a comprehensive review. *Clin Obstet Gynecol* 2007 Dec; 50(4): 868–77.

Zonderman, Jon, and Laurel Shader. *Birth Control Pills*. Chelsea House, 2006.

BREAST IMPLANTS

Breast implants are medical devices that are designed for women who want to increase their breast size (breast augmentation) or who need breast reconstruction (e.g., after mastectomy). Implants typically consist of a silicone elastomer shell that is filled with silicone gel or saline. Saline-filled implants have silicone shells that are either prefilled or filled during surgery, which allows for adjustments in size. Silicone gel-filled implants have silicone shells that are prefilled with silicone gel. Breast implants vary in size, profile, and the type of surface (textured or smooth). As of 2008, there were four Food and Drug Administration–approved breast implants available. The two saline-filled implants are approved for augmentation in women eighteen years or older, while the two silicone gel-filled implants are approved for women twenty-two years or older. All the implants are approved for breast reconstruction in women of any age.

HOW TO PREPARE

Whether you are planning breast augmentation or breast reconstruction, the presurgical planning and consultation stage is critical. This is the time to choose a surgeon, check credentials, and establish open communication. The surgeon will evaluate your general health and risk factors and discuss the most appropriate type of breast implant, details of the surgery, and what to expect after surgery. You should express your expectations and weigh the risks and benefits of your decision. Some of the following facts about breast implants should be part of your decision making.

- Breast implants do not last forever. You will probably need one or more surgeries on your breasts to deal with complications or cosmetic problems.

- If you have your implants replaced, your risk of complications increases compared with your first surgery.

- Routine mammograms are more difficult when you have breast implants.

- If you want to breast-feed, breast implants may reduce or eliminate your milk production.

- For silicone-gel-filled implants, rupture is a possibility. Because ruptures may not produce symptoms, you should have an MRI three years after your implant surgery and every two years thereafter.

HOW IT IS DONE

The methods for inserting and positioning breast implants depend on your body structure and your doctor's recommendations. The incisions are made to be as inconspicuous as possible—under the armpit, under the breast, or around the areola. The surgeon lifts the breast tissue around the incision, inserts the implant, and then centers it under the nipple either above or under the pectoral muscle.

Postsurgical recovery is usually twenty-four to forty-eight hours, and you should restrict your activities for a few additional days. Most patients experience swelling and soreness for several weeks. Your physician will let you know when you can resume your regular activities and exercise program.

BENEFITS

Improved self-esteem, better-fitting clothes, and more self-confidence are some of the benefits women report after having breast implants. Women who have had a mastectomy often feel insecure about their sexuality and femininity, and having breast reconstruction can be very healing both physically and emotionally.

RISKS/SIDE EFFECTS

Like any surgical procedure, breast implantation poses a risk of infection, pain, swelling, bleeding, and the effects of anesthesia. Risks and side effects specifically associated with breast implants include the following:

- **Loss of sensation in the nipple and/or breast area.**

- **Inability to get an accurate mammogram.** Breast implants may block the view of tumors or other growths.

- **Inability to breast-feed.** Although many women who have breast implants are able to breast-feed, some are not.

- **Rupture.** Many ruptures are the result of natural aging of the device, trauma to the breast, or excessive compression to the breast. Rupture due to mammography is very rare but can occur.

- **Capsular contracture.** When the scar tissue or capsule that forms around the breast implant tightens and squeezes it, you have capsular contracture. Symptoms range from mild firmness and discomfort to severe pain, a distorted breast, and/or movement of the breast implant. Surgery may be necessary if the symptoms are severe.

READ MORE ABOUT IT

Bruning, Nancy. *Breast Implants: Everything You Need to Know.* Hunter House, 2002.

Tebbetts, John B., and Terrye B. Tebetts. *The Best Breast 2: The Ultimate Discriminating Woman's Resource for Breast Augmentation.* Brown Books, 2008.

Breast Enlargement. *See* "Breast Implants."

Breast Reconstruction. *See* "Breast Implants."

BREAST REDUCTION

Also known as reduction mammaplasty, this procedure removes excess breast fat, skin, and glandular tissue to achieve a breast size that is in proportion with your body and that makes you feel more self-confident and comfortable with your appearance. This procedure also achieves another very important goal for many women: it can relieve the posture problems and the back, neck, and shoulder pain associated with having very heavy, pendulous breasts. According to the American Society of Plastic Surgeons, more than 104,000 breast reduction surgeries were performed in 2006.

HOW IT IS DONE

Surgeons use different breast reduction techniques, but the most common one involves making an incision that goes around the areola, down the breast toward the crease between the breast and the abdomen, and then horizontally in the crease under the breast. Excess breast tissue, fat, and skin are removed to reduce the size of the breast.

In most women, the surgeon can allow the nipple and areola to remain attached to the breast. If your breasts are very large and pendulous, however, the surgeon may need to remove the nipple and areola and reattach them as a skin graft. This causes permanent loss of sensation and may also result in an inability to breast-feed.

HOW TO PREPARE

During your initial visit with the plastic surgeon you have chosen for your procedure, you should discuss your concerns and learn all about the procedure so you feel comfortable with both the surgeon and your decision to get breast reduction. During this visit your surgeon should:

- Explain the breast reduction surgery in detail and the expected results, including likely scarring

- Ask about your expectations for breast appearance after the surgery

- Examine and photograph your breasts for insurance preapproval and for reference during and after surgery

- Discuss factors that may affect the outcome of your surgery, including your age, skin condition, and the size and shape of your breasts

- Discuss the positioning of the nipple and areola

- Determine where the surgery will be performed—at an outpatient facility or in the hospital

Depending on your age, or if there is a history of breast cancer in your family, your surgeon may recommend a baseline mammogram before surgery and another mammogram several months postsurgery so he or she will be better able to detect any future changes in your breast tissue. If you smoke, you will be asked to stop several weeks before surgery. You should also stop taking aspirin and anti-inflammatory drugs at least one week before surgery. Breast reduction surgery is sometimes done on an outpatient basis. If this is the case for you, have someone drive you home and stay with you for several days.

BENEFITS

Women who have had breast reduction surgery report a wide range of benefits, from relief from back and neck pain to better posture, being able to buy "normal" clothing, feeling self-assured and feminine, and being able to participate in activities they could not take part in before (e.g., jogging, playing tennis, swimming). Some even say they can sleep and breathe easier.

RISKS/SIDE EFFECTS

Possible complications from breast reduction surgery include infection, bleeding, or reaction to the anesthesia. Pain is usually moderate and treatable with medication prescribed by your surgeon. The surgery may cause some nerve damage or reduce blood supply to the breast or the nipple, resulting in temporary or permanent loss of sensation in the breast, nipple, or both. Breast-feeding may not be possible after surgery.

READ MORE ABOUT IT

Polynice, Alain, and Aloysius Smith. *Your Complete Guide to Breast Reduction and Breast Lifts.* Addicus Books, 2006.

Snodgrass, Bethanne. *When Less Is More: The Complete Guide for Women Considering Breast Reduction Surgery.* Harper-Collins, 2005.

BREAST SELF-EXAMINATION (BSE)

Breast self-examination (BSE) is an easy technique women can do themselves to monitor their breast health. The American Cancer Society recommends that beginning in their twenties, women should become familiar with how their breasts look and feel normally so they can report any changes to their health care professional. Early detection of a breast lump—which in many cases is *not* cancerous—allows women to get timely treatment, if needed, or to be aware of benign growths that they can monitor with their doctor's guidance.

HOW TO PREPARE
Choose a convenient time the same time each month to do your BSE. The best time is about one week after the start of your period, which is when your breasts are least likely to be swollen or tender. If you are pregnant or nursing, your breasts may feel more lumpy than normal.

HOW IT IS DONE
Here is a step-by-step introduction to breast self-examination, based on the American Cancer Society guidelines:

- Disrobe from the waist up and lie down, placing your right arm behind your head.

- Using the finger pads of your three middle fingers on

your left hand, make overlapping, dime-sized circular motions to feel for lumps in your breast.

• Apply light pressure to feel the tissue closest to the skin, medium pressure to feel deeper, and firm pressure to feel the tissue closest to the ribs and chest. Use each type of pressure in an area before moving on to the next spot. Move around the breast in an up-and-down pattern starting at an imaginary line drawn straight down your side from under your arm and moving across the breast to the middle of your chest. Explore the entire breast until you feel only ribs as you travel down and your collarbone as you travel up.

• Repeat the examination on your left breast, using the finger pads of your right hand.

• Stand in front of a mirror and press down firmly on your hips with your hands. Look at your breasts for any changes in color, size, shape, dimpling, or scaliness of the nipple or skin.

• Examine under each arm with your arm only slightly raised. Raising your arm too high tightens the tissue and makes it hard to examine properly.

BENEFITS

When you know how your breasts feel normally, it is easier to detect any subtle but potentially serious changes. If you do BSE regularly—every month or every other month—you should be able to identify any changes quickly and see your doctor. Although most breast lumps that women find when doing BSE are not cancerous, some are. Doing regular BSEs allows you to find cancers at an early stage, when prompt treatment can save your life. Thus it is important to do BSEs monthly, especially if you are at increased risk of breast cancer.

RISKS/SIDE EFFECTS

Although BSEs are an important screening tool for breast cancer and other breast abnormalities, they are not perfect: such exams can miss tumors, as can other screening methods. That's why it's important to rely on more than one method when you are screening for breast cancer. Breast self-exams can also be challenging for women who have normally lumpy or dense breasts. Many women complain that they have "cottage cheese" breasts and that they can't tell "a lump from a clump." It may be helpful to ask your health care provider to evaluate your breast self-exam technique and help you make better use of this important screening tool.

READ MORE ABOUT IT

Knutson D, Steiner E. Screening for breast cancer: current recommendations and future directions. *Am Fam Physician* 2007 Jun 1; 75(11): 1660–66.

Tu SP et al. Breast self-examination: self-reported frequency, quality, and associated outcomes. *J Cancer Educ* 2006 Fall; 21(3): 175–81.

CESAREAN SECTION

A cesarean section (or C-section) is the delivery of an infant through an incision in the mother's belly and uterus. Since the 1960s, the rate of cesarean sections has risen dramatically from about 1 in every 20 live births to about 1 out of 4. This increase has led many experts to say that C-sections are being done more than needed and should be restricted to medical reasons only.

Indeed, most doctors perform C-sections because of difficulties that arise during labor or because of problems that are known in advance. Some of the medical reasons for performing a C-section include the following:

- Labor is hard, is slow, or stops completely.

- The infant is too large to be delivered through the birth canal.

- The infant shows signs of distress, such as a very slow or very fast heart rate.

- There is a problem with the umbilical cord (e.g., it is wrapped around the infant's neck) or with the placenta that puts the infant at risk.

- The infant is not in a head-down position.

- You have a heart condition that could be made worse by the stress of labor.

- You have an infection that could pass to your infant from the birth canal.

- You have a multiple birth.

- You are physically unable to bear down sufficiently to give birth vaginally.

- You have a history of cesarean section and your doctor thinks labor may rupture your previous scar.

HOW TO PREPARE

Cesarean sections can be planned (e.g., as when there is a known difficulty such as an infection that could pass to the child) or chosen when a situation arises during labor that requires the procedure. In either case, you will receive either spinal or epidural anesthesia to numb your belly and legs. You may also receive a sedative to help you relax. General anesthesia is typically used only in an emergency.

HOW IT IS DONE

Once your belly and legs are numb, the physician makes an incision, usually just above the pubic hair line. This is sometimes referred to as a "bikini cut." In some cases the incision is made from the navel down to the pubic area. Once the doctor lifts the infant out and removes the placenta, the incision is closed with stitches.

BENEFITS

The benefits of cesarean section relate to the reasons it needs to be done for medical reasons. For example, if you have a heart condition, it prevents undue stress that could be harmful or life-threatening; if your infant was positioned in a way that made vaginal delivery impossible, it could save your infant's life.

RISKS/SIDE EFFECTS

A C-section is major surgery and so has some possible risks, including:

- Heavy blood loss

- Infection of the uterus or the incision

- Injury to the infant or mother

- Blood clots in your legs

- Side effects from the anesthesia, such as nausea, vomiting, and severe headache

Most women stay in the hospital for three to five days after having a C-section, and then it takes about a month or longer to fully recover. You can expect vaginal bleeding for several weeks (use pads, not tampons) and pain in the lower belly for one to two weeks. You should avoid lifting and doing vigorous exercise until your incision heals completely. If you notice any pus or red streaks at your incision site and/or you experience a fever, you should call your physician immediately.

READ MORE ABOUT IT

Connolly, Maureen, and Dana Sullivan. *The Essential C-Section Guide: Pain Control, Healing at Home, Getting Your Body Back, and Everything Else You Need to Know About a Cesarean Birth.* Broadway, 2004.

Moore, Michele C., and Caroline M. de Costa. *Cesarean Section: Understanding and Celebrating Your Baby's Birth.* Johns Hopkins University Press, 2003.

CHEMOTHERAPY

The strict definition of chemotherapy is any treatment that uses chemical substances or drugs, but today the word has come to mean drugs used to treat cancer. Chemotherapy is a systemic treatment, which means that it enters the bloodstream and affects the entire body. The goal of chemotherapy is to destroy any cancer cells that have spread from where the cancer started in the body.

Although each type of cancer affects the body in different ways, all cancers have at least one thing in common: they involve abnormal cells that, for some reason, grow out of control. This similarity among cancers, however, is not enough to make it possible to treat every cancer patient with the same chemotherapy. Your doctor will decide which drug or combination of drugs best fits your needs.

HOW TO PREPARE
Your body's response to chemotherapy will depend on the type of drug(s) you are given, your overall health status, and how well you prepare for treatment. Here are a few suggestions:

- Ask your oncologist what side effects to expect.

- Plan to have someone drive you to and from your appointments.

- Get help at home with chores such as shopping, cooking, and cleaning while you are undergoing chemotherapy.

- Stock up on soft foods to eat during your treatment.
  Applesauce, bananas, mashed potatoes, oatmeal, soft-
  boiled eggs, and yogurt are good choices.

HOW IT WORKS

The reason anticancer drugs work is because they are designed to interfere with the activity of cancer cells, many of
which divide rapidly, and some of which reproduce more
slowly. However, chemotherapy also affects healthy cells,
which results in a variety of side effects in different parts of
the body (see "Risks/Side Effects"). For example, chemotherapy that eliminates fast-growing cancer cells also destroys
other fast-growing cells, which include blood and hair cells.

Chemotherapy can be taken as a pill or liquid; it can be
administered in your doctor's office, in a hospital, or at a clinic
as a shot, or it can be given intravenously. It can be taken daily,
once a week, or even once a month, depending on the type of
cancer you have and the chemotherapy you are taking. (See
"Chemotherapy Drugs" in Part III.)

BENEFITS

Each person who receives chemotherapy reacts to and benefits from it in her own way. Chemotherapy can reduce the risk
of recurrence, improve quality of life, relieve symptoms, and
extend survival.

A good example of the benefits of chemotherapy can be
seen in the Early Breast Cancer Trialists' Collaborative Group
(EBCTCG) study, which reported its findings in the May 14,
2005, issue of *Lancet.* The EBCTCG analyzed data from 194
studies that included 145,000 women who had early-stage
breast cancer. The women received chemotherapy, hormone
therapy, or chemotherapy plus hormone therapy. The investigators looked at the effects of chemotherapy and hormone therapy after fifteen years. Chemotherapy included

CMF (cyclophosphamide, methotrexate, and fluorouracil), anthracycline-based chemotherapy combinations such as FAC (fluorouracil, doxorubicin, and cyclophosphamide), or FEC (fluorouracil, epirubicin, and cyclophosphamide); tamoxifen was the hormonal therapy.

The findings were impressive. Six months of anthracycline-based chemotherapy improved the survival rate in women younger than fifty by 38 percent and in women fifty to sixty-nine by 20 percent compared to women who did not have chemotherapy. The investigators also found that anthracycline-based chemotherapy was significantly more effective than CMF chemotherapy. When they looked at tamoxifen, women with estrogen-receptor-positive cancer who took tamoxifen for five years had a significantly improved survival rate of 31 percent compared with similar women who did not take tamoxifen. Five years of tamoxifen also significantly improved survival and reduced recurrence compared with women who took it for only one to two years.

Overall, the researchers found that six months of anthracycline-based chemotherapy followed by five years of tamoxifen improved survival rates by about 50 percent in women younger than fifty who had early-stage, estrogen-receptor-positive breast cancer, which is the most common type of breast cancer. In older women (fifty to sixty-nine years) with the same type of cancer, the same treatment plan improved survival rates by about 40 percent. In both situations, the benefits were compared with those of women who had not received chemotherapy or tamoxifen.

RISKS/SIDE EFFECTS
Chemotherapy drugs can cause a wide variety of side effects, depending on the drug taken. Nausea and vomiting are common reactions to many chemotherapy drugs, as are loss of libido, mouth sores, hair loss, diarrhea, fatigue, dry skin, easy bruising, and easy bleeding. Fortunately, there are many treatments available to help alleviate or prevent side effects of chemotherapy.

READ MORE ABOUT IT
Early Breast Cancer Trialists' Collaborative Group. Effects of chemotherapy and hormonal therapy for early breast cancer on recurrence and 15-year survival: an overview of the randomised trials. *Lancet* 2005 May 14–20; 365(9472): 1687–717.

Lyss, Alan P., Humberto Fagundes, and Patricia Corrigan. *Chemotherapy and Radiation for Dummies*. For Dummies, 2005.

Skeel, Roland T. *Handbook of Cancer Chemotherapy*. Lippincott, Williams & Wilkins, 2007.

COLPOSCOPY

If your Pap test results come back showing abnormal cell growth, your doctor will probably order a colposcopy. A colposcopy is a procedure that allows a health care professional to closely examine your cervix with a colposcope, an instrument that magnifies the surface of the cervix and vagina ten to forty times, to uncover the source of the abnormal cells. The presence of abnormal cells does not always mean cervical cancer. In fact, a vaginal infection, such as human papillomavirus, is often the culprit.

HOW TO PREPARE
Having a colposcopy requires minimal preparation. Schedule the procedure for a time you will not be having your period, as the test cannot be done accurately during that time. Also, for twenty-four hours before the colposcopy do not have sexual intercourse or use douches, tampons, or any type of vaginal creams, powders, or medications.

Before the procedure, you should empty your bladder and bowels, as this will help make you feel more comfortable during the exam. Many physicians recommend that you take an over-the-counter pain reliever one hour before the procedure to help alleviate any discomfort you may feel.

HOW IT IS DONE

Having a colposcopy is similar to having a pelvic examination and Pap test. While you are on the table with your feet in the stirrups, a doctor will insert a speculum into your vagina. This holds your vagina open so your doctor can see your cervix. The doctor will position the colposcope (a lighted microscope) so he or she can look into your vagina. The doctor will clean your cervix with a saline solution and then apply a vinegar solution (acetic acid) with a cotton swab. Acetic acid reacts differently when it makes contact with abnormal tissue versus normal tissue. If the acetic acid doesn't show any abnormalities, another substance called Lugol's solution can be used to identify abnormal cells.

If your doctor sees abnormal tissue, he or she can increase the magnification of the colposcope to identify more characteristics of the tissue. Your doctor may also choose to do a biopsy.

BENEFITS

Colposcopy is a simple, accurate screening tool for detection of cervical, uterine, and vulvar cancers. Early detection of such cancers will allow you to get immediate treatment and could save your life. In many cases, however, a colposcopy uncovers an infection, and that, too, can be treated promptly before it could possibly cause serious problems.

RISKS/SIDE EFFECTS

Colposcopy is associated with little to no risk. You may experience bleeding after the procedure, and there is a very slight risk of infection. If you experience any of the following after the procedure, see your doctor immediately:

- Excessive vaginal bleeding (using more than one sanitary pad an hour)

- Fever higher than 100.4°F

- Thick, yellowish vaginal discharge and/or foul-smelling vaginal odor

READ MORE ABOUT IT

Martin JT. Do women comply with recommendations for Papanicolaou smears following colposcopy? A retrospective study. *J Midwifery Womens Health* 2008 Mar–Apr; 53(2): 138–42.

Pruitt SL et al. Communicating colposcopy results: what do patients and providers discuss? *J Low Genit Tract Dis* 2008 Apr; 12(2): 95–102.

CRYOSURGERY

Cryosurgery (also called cryotherapy) is a method that uses extreme cold to kill abnormal cells and tumors, both external and internal. For our purposes, we look at cryosurgery of the cervix, which is most often done to destroy abnormal cervical cells that show changes (cervical dysplasia) that may result in cancer. Cryosurgery for breast tumors is still in the research stage.

Cryosurgery is usually done after a colposcopy has established the existence of abnormal cervical cells, but it is also used to treat cervicitis (inflammation of the cervix).

HOW TO PREPARE

Cryosurgery requires virtually no preparation. You may take a pain reliever (e.g., ibuprofen) an hour or so before the procedure to help eliminate cramping and pain. You should not schedule the procedure for when you are menstruating.

HOW IT IS DONE

Cryosurgery is done in your doctor's office and begins similar to a pelvic exam: you lie on an exam table with your feet in stirrups, and the clinician inserts a speculum into your vagina so your cervix can be seen. This is when the actual freezing portion of the surgery begins.

The clinician inserts special instruments called cryo-probes into your vagina until they cover the abnormal tissue. Liquid nitrogen flows through the cryoprobes, which causes them to freeze and destroy superficial abnormal cervical tissue.

To get the most effective results, the area should be treated for three minutes, allowed to thaw, and then treated again for three minutes.

BENEFITS

Cryosurgery is minimally invasive, as it involves only a small incision or insertion of the cryoprobe through the skin. This minimizes pain, bleeding, and any other complications associated with surgery. As a result, recovery time and hospital stay (if one is needed at all) are very short. In some cases, the procedure can be done using only local anesthesia.

Clinicians can focus cryosurgical treatment to a limited area and thus avoid destroying nearby healthy tissue. Cryo-surgery can be repeated safely and used along with standard treatments, such as radiation, hormone therapy, chemotherapy, and surgery. Patients who are not good candidates for conventional surgery usually can tolerate cryosurgery. For individuals who have inoperable cancer or cancer that has not responded to standard treatments, cryosurgery is an option.

RISKS/SIDE EFFECTS

Cervical cryosurgery can cause cramping, bleeding, or pain, but it has not been shown to have a negative impact on fertility. For several weeks after the procedure, you may experience a watery discharge, which contains dead cervical tissue. If, however, you experience fever, heavy bleeding, severe pelvic pain, or a foul-smelling vaginal discharge, contact your doctor immediately.

After cryosurgery, you will need to have a Pap test every three to six months. Once you have had several consecutive normal Pap smears, you and your physician can determine how often you need to have subsequent Pap tests.

READ MORE ABOUT IT

Luciani S et al. Effectiveness of cryotherapy treatment for cervical intraepithelial neoplasia. *Int J Gynaecol Obstet* 2008 May; 101(2): 172–77.

Persad VL et al. Management of cervical neoplasia: a 13-year experience with cryotherapy and laser. *J Low Genit Tract Dis* 2001 Oct; 5(4): 199–203.

DIAPHRAGM

A diaphragm is a soft rubber dome-shaped device that covers the cervix and thus prevents sperm from entering the uterus. It is often referred to as a barrier method of birth control. A diaphragm is used along with a spermicide, a gel-like substance that kills any sperm that may get past the protective barrier.

Studies show that when a diaphragm and spermicide are used correctly and consistently, the failure rate is approximately 5 percent; that means out of 100 women who use this birth control method, 5 will become pregnant. In reality, the failure rate is approximately 18 to 20 percent, because some women and their partners do not use this method correctly.

HOW IT IS USED

To work effectively, the diaphragm needs to be inserted correctly along with a spermicide before each sexual intercourse encounter. Here are some guidelines for correct use:

- Spread spermicidal jelly or cream inside the dome of the diaphragm and around the rim before you insert it.

- Fold the diaphragm in half, making sure the jelly or cream stays inside. Insert the diaphragm all the way into the vagina so that it covers the cervix. Tuck the forward rim of the diaphragm up behind the pelvic bone (the bone that forms the front of the pelvis) and the back rim up behind the cervix.

- Insert the diaphragm no more than six hours before having sexual intercourse.

- Leave the diaphragm in for six to eight hours after intercourse. If you have intercourse again within this time, you do not have to remove the diaphragm: just insert more spermicide into your vagina.

- Do not leave the diaphragm in for more than twenty-four hours because there is a risk of toxic shock syndrome.

- After you remove the diaphragm, wash it with warm water and hand soap. Dry it thoroughly and store it in its container.

- Check the diaphragm regularly for holes by holding it up to a light and stretching the rubber.

- If you have any problems inserting the diaphragm, contact your physician or health care professional for instructions.

BENEFITS
The benefits of using a diaphragm are that it is reusable, small, and easy to carry; it rarely affects sexual arousal or experience; and it is relatively inexpensive.

RISKS/SIDE EFFECTS
The most common side effect associated with using a diaphragm is irritation of the vaginal tissues. If you have a latex allergy, history of toxic shock syndrome, or abnormalities of

the cervix or vagina, you could also experience some problems with using a diaphragm.

READ MORE ABOUT IT
Kass-Annese, Barbara, and Hal C. Danzer. *Natural Birth Control Made Simple.* Hunter House, 2003.

DILATATION AND CURETTAGE (D&C)

Dilatation and curettage (D&C) is a surgical procedure in which a metal instrument called a curette is used to scrape the lining of the uterus. In past decades, D&C was performed mainly to help diagnose the cause of abnormal uterine bleeding. It is still done for that purpose today, although now it is often used along with other procedures, including hysteroscopy and polypectomy. Dilatation and curettage is also frequently done to complete a miscarriage or an abortion.

HOW TO PREPARE
If you are scheduled for a D&C, avoid all food and beverages, including water, for at least seven hours before the operation. You may also be asked to stop taking aspirin and other nonsteroidal anti-inflammatory drugs for seven days prior to surgery.

HOW IT IS DONE
A D&C is performed in a hospital or, in some cases, a specially designated room in a doctor's office. After you are positioned on the table with your feet in stirrups and you receive anesthesia, the physician will clean your cervix and vagina with an antibacterial scrub. An instrument is used to gradually widen the opening to the uterus, and when it has reached the desired size, the curette (an instrument with a flat metal

loop at the end) is inserted into the uterus and used to scrape the lining until all the desired tissue has been removed.

BENEFITS
Women who have a D&C have a lower rate of unplanned hospital admissions than women who have miscarriages either with or without medical intervention. When a D&C is done for a miscarriage, it also allows for testing to be done to find a possible cause of the lost pregnancy.

RISKS/SIDE EFFECTS
Most women go home the same day after the D&C has been done. Backache and mild cramps are common side effects, along with the passing of small blood clots for a day or so. Spotting may continue for several weeks. Patients should avoid douching, tampons, and sexual intercourse for at least two weeks postsurgery.

The most common complication associated with a D&C is puncture or perforation of the uterus with one of the surgical instruments. Although this sounds serious, unless internal organs or large blood vessels are damaged, such holes nearly always heal themselves. Other risks include infection (indications include fever, heavy bleeding, severe cramps, foul-smelling vaginal discharge) and bleeding. Physicians who believe there is a risk of infection often prescribe antibiotics both before and after the procedure. This is especially important in patients who have certain heart defects, as the antibiotics can help prevent vaginal bacteria from infecting the heart valves.

READ MORE ABOUT IT
Fauci, Anthony S et al. *Harrison's Principles of Internal Medicine.* 17th edition. McGraw-Hill Professional, 2008.

DOUCHING

The French have given us the word *douche,* which means to wash or soak. Douching refers to washing or cleaning out the vagina with water or a combination of fluids, many of which can be purchased premixed at drug and grocery stores. Common ingredients are water along with vinegar, baking soda, or iodine, packaged in a bottle that has a tube or nozzle through which the fluid can be squirted into the vagina. Some women prepare their own douches using herbs.

It is estimated that 20 to 40 percent of women ages fifteen to forty-four douche regularly, and that about half of them douche every week. Their reasons include wanting to clean the vagina and/or clean away any residual menstrual blood, getting rid of odors, avoiding sexually transmitted diseases, and preventing pregnancy.

In fact, none of these is a valid reason to douche. The best way to clean the vagina is to let nature take its course: it cleans itself. You should use mild soap and water to keep your genital area clean, but cleaning inside your vagina is not necessary. If you douche to get rid of vaginal odors, it will only cover up the smell. If your vagina has a foul odor, this could be a sign of a bacterial infection, sexually transmitted disease, urinary tract infection, or other infection, and you should consult your doctor as soon as possible to eliminate the cause of the odor.

RISKS/SIDE EFFECTS

The consensus among most experts, including those associated with the American College of Obstetricians and Gynecologists, is that douching is not a healthy habit and should be avoided. That's because douching can quickly change the delicate balance of bacterial flora in the vagina, which then makes women more likely to get vaginal infections and possibly spread existing infections up into the uterus, fallopian tubes, and ovaries.

Many women douche to get rid of vaginal pain, itching, burning, or discharge, but they do not realize that douching actually makes these problems worse. Research shows that women who douche regularly have more health problems than women who do not. Those problems include vaginal irritation, sexually transmitted diseases, pelvic inflammatory disease, and bacterial vaginosis.

If you think that douching can help prevent STDs or pregnancy, think again. In fact, douching may actually make it easier to get pregnant because it can push the sperm farther up into the vagina and cervix. Douching also is not a way to prevent STDs.

READ MORE ABOUT IT

Cottrell BH. Discussing the health risks of douching. *AWHONN Lifelines* 2006 Apr–May; 10(2): 130–36.

Hutchinson KB et al. Vaginal douching and development of bacterial vaginosis among women with normal and abnormal vaginal microflora. *Sex Transm Dis* 2007 Sep; 34(9): 671–75.

ELECTROSURGICAL LOOP EXCISION (LEEP)

Electrosurgical loop excision (LEEP) is a procedure in which a thin, low-voltage electrified wire loop is used to cut out (excise) abnormal tissue. It is typically ordered after an abnormal Pap test results have been confirmed by colposcopy and cervical biopsy. At that point, LEEP can be used to remove abnormal cervical tissue.

HOW TO PREPARE
Generally, LEEP requires little or no preparation. You should schedule the procedure for when you are not having your period. Your doctor will explain the procedure to you and ask you to sign a consent form. You do not need to fast or take a sedative before the procedure. You should tell your doctor if you are pregnant; if you have allergies to any medications, latex, tape, iodine, or anesthetic agents; if you have a history of a bleeding disorder; and if you are taking herbal supplements, anticoagulant medications, aspirin, or other medications that affect blood clotting. You may be asked to stop taking any substances that affect blood clotting for one week before the procedure.

HOW IT IS DONE
Electrosurgical loop excision is usually done at a health professional's office, a clinic, or a hospital as an outpatient procedure. You will lie on an examining table with your feet in

stirrups. Similar to a pelvic exam, your clinician will insert a speculum into your vagina to gently spread apart the vaginal walls to allow your vagina and cervix to be examined. He or she may apply a vinegar or iodine solution to your cervix to make abnormal cells more visible. If your doctor plans to give you a cervical block (medication injected to numb the cervix), you will be given an oral or intravenous pain medication along with a local anesthetic.

A colposcope is placed near the opening of the vagina so your physician will have a magnified view of the cervix. Once your cervix is numb, your physician will pass the electrically charged loop through the speculum and up to the cervix. As the loop passes across the cervix, it cuts a thin layer of tissue that contains abnormal cells. A medicated paste is then applied to prevent bleeding.

The entire procedure takes fifteen to twenty minutes, and you can go home immediately after the procedure.

BENEFITS
LEEP is a very effective treatment for abnormal cervical cell changes, as effective as cryotherapy or laser treatment. If the clinician successfully removes all the abnormal tissue, no further surgery is needed, although it is possible that abnormal cells may develop in the future. Several studies show that all abnormal cells were removed in as many as 98 percent of cases.

RISKS/SIDE EFFECTS
Most women can return to their normal activities within one to three days after undergoing LEEP, with a few notable exceptions. On the "to avoid" list for the first three weeks after the procedure are the use of tampons and sexual intercourse. Douching should never be done.

Normal side effects after LEEP include mild cramping for several hours, a dark brown vaginal discharge during the first week, and vaginal discharge or spotting for about three weeks. Rarely, an infection of the cervix or uterus may develop or narrowing of the cervix can cause infertility. In less than

10 percent of women, excessive bleeding requires vaginal packing or a blood transfusion.

READ MORE ABOUT IT

Martin-Hirsch PL et al. Surgery for cervical intraepithelial neoplasia. *Cochrane Database of Systematic Reviews* 2000; (2): CD001318.

Nuovo J et al. Treatment outcomes for squamous intraepithelial lesions. *Intl J Gynecol Obstet* 2000; 68(1): 25–33.

Samson SA et al. The effect of loop electrosurgical excision procedure on future pregnancy outcomes. *Obstet Gynecol* 2005; 105(2): 325–32.

GYNECOLOGIC EXAMINATION

A gynecologic examination is a physical exam that focuses on the pelvic area (which is` why it is also called a pelvic exam) for the purpose of detecting any abnormalities and/or to treat existing conditions. It may be performed by a gynecologist or by a general or family practitioner, an internist, or by a nurse practitioner who specializes in this area. Physicians generally agree that women should get a gynecologic examination often, but there is no consensus on what "often" means. Most experts agree that the first checkup should occur in females between the ages of sixteen and nineteen or earlier if the girl has been sexually active at a younger age. After that time, some of the procedures that are part of the exam are recommended once a year, while others can be done every two or three years until age forty, when the recommendations change.

A thorough gynecologic examination includes taking a complete history, a physical examination, a pelvic examination, a rectovaginal and/or rectal examination (only for women of a certain age), laboratory tests (if needed), and a discussion with the doctor about the findings.

HOW TO PREPARE
Preparation for a gynecologic examination is simple:

- Schedule your appointment for when you will not have your period. If, however, you have new or increasing pelvic pain or new vaginal discharge, a pelvic exam can be done while you are menstruating.

• Do not use tampons, vaginal medications, vaginal sprays or powders, or douches for at least twenty-four hours before your appointment.

• Avoid having sexual intercourse for twenty-four hours before your exam if you have abnormal vaginal discharge.

For comfort, it is also best to empty your bladder before your exam if you will be undergoing an internal pelvic examination.

HOW IT IS DONE

There are some variations among physicians, but the general approach to a thorough gynecologic examination is as follows:

• **Complete history.** The physician will ask about your health history and that of your immediate family, including medication use, history of hospitalizations and illnesses, current complaints, menstrual history, birth control methods used (past and present), supplement use, and any adverse reactions to drugs.

• **Physical examination.** This includes measurement of height and weight, pulse, blood pressure, and temperature. Many physicians also examine the neck for thyroid enlargement and tender lymph nodes. The breasts should be examined for lumps, tenderness, dimpling, nipple discharge, and any other signs of a tumor.

• **Pelvic examination.** This takes place while you are lying on your back on an examining table with your feet in stirrups. The doctor will examine the external genital area and then do an internal exam. Depending on the physician and whether you are getting a Pap smear done, he or she may then insert a metal or plastic speculum into your vagina so the cervix and vaginal walls can be inspected. If a Pap smear is planned, it can be taken at this time. Several other examinations are often done while you are on the table.

- **A bimanual examination** may also be done, which involves the doctor inserting two fingers of one hand into the vagina and placing the other hand on your abdomen. This allows the clinician to check the position, mobility, firmness, and size of your uterus, locate the ovaries and fallopian tubes, and check the abdominal area for any abnormalities.

- **A rectovaginal examination,** during which the clinician keeps one finger in the vagina while inserting another into the rectum. This allows the doctor to check the wall between the rectum and vagina and to feel the pelvic organs.

- **A rectal examination,** usually done for women age fifty and older, in which the clinician inserts one finger into the rectum to check for growths or other abnormalities.

Laboratory tests that may be ordered include a urine test for protein, sugar, and blood; a Pap smear (as noted above); a gonorrhea culture (usually reserved for women who think they are at risk); a blood count for anemia; a test for syphilis; a test for vaginal infections; and a mammogram.

Once the examination is over, the clinician should discuss any findings and explain which tests were taken and when results can be expected.

BENEFITS
A gynecologic examination, especially when done regularly, allows you and your clinician to keep track of any changes

and to act in a timely manner if any abnormalities are found. Having this exam could literally save your life.

RISKS/SIDE EFFECTS
There are no risks or side effects associated with this examination.

READ MORE ABOUT IT
Chernecky, C. C., and B. J. Berger, eds. *Laboratory Tests and Diagnostic Procedures.* Saunders, 2004.

HORMONE REPLACEMENT THERAPY

Hormone replacement therapy is the use of medications that contain female hormones to replace the ones the body is no longer producing. The two main types of hormone therapy are:

- **Estrogen therapy** (ET), in which estrogen is taken alone. This approach is generally used only by women who no longer have a uterus.

- **Progesterone/progestin-estrogen therapy** (HRT), also called combination therapy, in which doses of estrogen and progesterone or progestin (synthetic progesterone) are given together in varying amounts. The two hormones are given together to prevent the overgrowth of the endometrium (the uterine lining). It is designed for women who have a uterus.

At one time, doctors routinely prescribed hormone replacement therapy for women to ease menopausal symptoms, most notably the hot flashes, mood swings, urinary difficulties, depression, and vaginal dryness that affect so many women. It was also believed to help prevent heart disease and osteoporosis. But when the 2002 Women's Health Initiative (WHI) trial reported that hormone therapy presented more health risks than benefits, up to two-thirds of women who were taking hormone therapy stopped, many without telling their doctors. They, and many of their doctors, were understandably alarmed and confused.

Today, confusion about hormone therapy continues, but research continues to add new information that can be helpful in deciding whether you should or need to take hormone therapy. One critical element is that the WHI used synthetic progestin and synthetic estrogen, not bioidentical hormones (which mimic the body's natural cycles)—a point that could explain, at least partly according to some experts, the dangers discovered with the use of synthetic hormone therapy. If you are considering hormone replacement therapy, it is good to know that you have a choice—conventional synthetic hormones or bioidentical hormones—and that it is important for you to talk with knowledgeable professionals about the pros and cons of both.

HOW IT IS DONE

The use of hormone replacement therapy is a highly individual decision, and one that should be made after consulting knowledgeable health care professionals about both synthetic and bioidentical hormones. The National Heart, Lung and Blood Institute (NHLBI) recommends that women who are thinking about hormone replacement therapy consider these guidelines:

- Do not start or continue hormone replacement therapy for the purpose of preventing heart disease. You should consider other prevention methods, especially lifestyle changes, rather than depend on hormone therapy.

- If you are worried about osteoporosis, consult your doctor and consider other options rather than hormone replacement therapy as preventive measures.

- Continue getting your routine mammograms and doing breast self-examinations regardless of whether you use hormone replacement therapy, but especially if you do.

- Talk to your doctor about your personal risks and benefits of using hormone replacement therapy.

Regarding the last suggestion by the NHLBI, here are some suggestions you can discuss with your health care provider on how to minimize the inherent risks of hormone therapy:

- **Timing is everything (or at least very important).** Recent studies suggest that the risk of hormone therapy causing heart disease is not significantly greater in women younger than age sixty. Some studies also indicate that estrogen may protect the heart if it is taken early in menopause, if indeed you begin menopause at or around the average age of fifty to fifty-four.

- **Keep it low.** Use the lowest effective dose for the least amount of time you need to treat your symptoms. (As an aside from NHLBI suggestions, you might want to investigate complementary ways—nutritional supplements, herbal remedies—to relieve those symptoms.)

- **Pick a delivery system.** Estrogen can be taken in the form of a pill, patch, gel, slow-release suppository or ring, or vaginal cream. Estrogen applied directly to your vagina is more effective at a lower dose than estrogen in a pill or as a patch. This form may be best if you are experiencing only isolated vaginal symptoms. If you have not had a hysterectomy and are using the pill or patch form of estrogen, you will need to balance it with progestin, which is available in a pill, combination pill, vaginal gel, combination skin patch, or intrauterine device. You and your physician should discuss which approach is best for you.

BENEFITS

Estrogen is an effective treatment for relief of hot flashes, night sweats, and vaginal symptoms of menopause, including itching, burning, dryness, and discomfort with intercourse.

Several studies conducted since the WHI study (one in 2006 in the *Journal of Women's Health* and another in 2006 in the *Archives of Internal Medicine*) found that estrogen may reduce the risk of heart disease when given to younger women, at the onset of menopause, rather than in older women. Hormone therapy can also help prevent bone loss and decreases the risk of colorectal cancer.

If you are considering bioidentical hormones, one of the biggest benefits of this form of hormone therapy is that it is individualized: while synthetic hormone therapy comes in prepackaged formulations determined by the pharmaceutical companies, bioidentical hormones are formulated specifically for you by a compounding pharmacist to match your body's needs. Another benefit is that the body can metabolize bioidentical hormones as it was designed to do, which minimizes the risk of side effects. Synthetic hormones are foreign substances and often produce intolerable side effects.

RISKS/SIDE EFFECTS

The WHI found that women who were taking the synthetic combination of estrogen and progestin (Prempro) had an increased risk of developing heart disease (by 24 percent), breast cancer, stroke (41 percent), and blood clots. For example, daily use of this combination of hormones increases your chance of developing breast cancer by about 5 to 6 percent with each year you take the hormones. Therefore, if you took HRT for ten years, your risk of breast cancer would be 50 to 60 percent higher than it was before you started therapy. This finding has been seen in the WHI study and many other studies.

Another finding of the WHI was that HRT slightly increased a woman's risk of Alzheimer's disease rather than protected against it. Yet another discovery was that women who were taking this combination of hormones had an increase in abnormal mammograms, specifically a higher number of false positives. This is believed to be caused by the estrogen, which increases breast tissue density. Use of estrogen without progestin also increases the risk of uterine (endo-metrial) cancer.

Women who take estrogen replacement therapy have a higher risk for ovarian cancer compared with women who do not take hormones after menopause. This risk increases the longer you use estrogen and is especially high among those who have used it for more than ten years. The WHI found only a possible slightly increased risk of ovarian cancer in women who use HRT.

READ MORE ABOUT IT

PM Medical Health News. *21st Century Complete Medical Guide to Menopause, Premature Ovarian Failure (POV), Hormone Replacement Therapy, Estrogen Therapy: Authoritative Federal Government Clinical Data and Practical Information for Patients and Physicians*. CD-ROM. Progressive Management, 2004.

Ribot C, Tremollieres F. Hormone replacement therapy in postmenopausal women: all the treatments are not the same. *Gynecol Obstet Fertil* 2007 May; 35(5): 388–97.

Rosenthal, M. Sara. *The Natural Woman's Guide to Hormone Replacement Therapy: An Alternative Approach*. New Page Books, 2003.

The Writing Group for the WHI Investigators. Risks and benefits of estrogen plus progestin in healthy post-menopausal women: Principal results of the Women's Health Initiative randomized controlled trial. *JAMA* 2002; 288(3): 321–33.

The Women's Health Initiative Steering Committee. Effects of conjugated equine estrogen in postmenopausal women with hysterectomy. The Women's Health Initiative Randomized Controlled Trial. *JAMA* 2004; 291:1701–12.

HYSTERECTOMY

Hysterectomy is the surgical removal of the uterus. It is the second most common major operation performed in the United States, second only to cesarean section. Approximately 600,000 American women undergo the procedure every year. By age sixty, one-third of the women in the United States have had a hysterectomy.

Although there is much debate about the number of unnecessary hysterectomies that are performed each year, there are also many necessary and serious indications for having it done.

- **Gynecologic cancer.** Hysterectomy is often the treatment chosen for cancer of the uterus or cervix, depending on how advanced the disease is and the specific type of cancer involved.

- **Fibroids.** Hysterectomy is the only permanent way to deal with fibroids. However, since many women with fibroids have mild symptoms, hysterectomy should be reserved for only the more serious cases.

- **Endometriosis.** If medication and conservative methods don't improve symptoms of endometriosis, hysterectomy may be an appropriate option (see "Endometriosis" in Part I).

- **Uterine prolapse.** If other medical options don't adequately correct problems associated with uterine prolapse, which can include urinary incontinence and problems with bowel movements, hysterectomy may be necessary (see "Prolapsed Uterus" in Part I).

- **Persistent vaginal bleeding.** If your periods are heavy and irregular and bleeding can't be controlled by nonsurgical approaches, hysterectomy can be considered.

Because hysterectomy ends the ability to become pregnant, it's important that you discuss other treatment options with your doctor if you think or know you want to become pregnant. Although a hysterectomy may be the only viable option when cancer is involved, the other conditions may respond adequately to alternative treatments.

HOW TO PREPARE
Pack your bags, because hysterectomy is an inpatient procedure. The length of your hospital stay will depend on the type of hysterectomy you have, your doctor's recommendations, and how quickly you recover. Generally, abdominal hysterectomy requires a one-to-two-day hospital stay. Once you get home, however, you will need several weeks to recover completely, and so you should arrange to have some help with housework, shopping, child care, lifting, and other activities that could set back your recovery or even injure you.

HOW IT IS DONE
The vast majority of these procedures are abdominal hysterectomies, which means the surgeon makes an incision in your lower abdomen through which he or she removes the uterus; one or both ovaries and fallopian tubes can also be removed if necessary. An alternative procedure is a vaginal hysterectomy, which is done through an incision in the vagina. The abdominal procedure is preferred, however, if you have a

large uterus or if your doctor plans to check other pelvic organs for disease. In either case, the procedure is done under general anesthesia and lasts about one to two hours.

Before the procedure begins, a member of your surgical team will introduce a catheter through your urethra to empty your bladder. The catheter will remain in place throughout the surgery and for a short time afterward. Someone will also clean your abdomen and vagina with a sterile solution and shave the incision site.

Once you have received anesthesia, your surgeon will make the incision in your lower abdomen to reach your uterus. The incision will be one of two types: a vertical incision that starts in the middle of your abdomen and extends from just below your navel to just above your pubic bone, or a horizontal bikini-line incision that lies about one inch above your pubic bone. The choice of incision depends on the size of your uterus, if you have any scars from previous surgeries, and the need to explore other organs in the area for signs of disease.

In some cases, another procedure called a salpingo-oophorectomy (removal of one or both ovaries [bilateral] and the fallopian tubes) is done at the same time as the hysterectomy (see "Miscellaneous Invasive Procedures").

After surgery, you'll remain in the recovery room for several hours and be monitored for signs of pain. You'll be given medication for pain and to prevent infection. Most women are up and walking the next day and well enough to go home in another day or two.

BENEFITS
For some women, the fact that they will not have to worry about getting pregnant is a benefit; for others it is not. The lack of menstrual periods, however, is usually welcome. Some women report an increase in sexual pleasure, which may be due to the elimination of chronic pelvic pain, cramping, or fear of pregnancy.

RISKS/SIDE EFFECTS

You will need to use sanitary pads for the bloody vaginal drainage and bleeding that normally occurs for several days after a hysterectomy. Your doctor will tell you to restrict your physical activities, especially lifting, for six weeks or longer, depending on the extent of your surgery. Most women can resume sexual activity six weeks after surgery.

As with any surgery, there is a risk of blood clots, severe infection, adhesions, bowel obstruction, or postoperative hemorrhage, although hysterectomy has a very low surgical risk level. Some women develop a mild bladder or wound infection, which can usually be treated with antibiotics.

READ MORE ABOUT IT

Parkinson-Hardman, Linda. *101 Handy Hints for a Happy Hysterectomy.* Lulu.com, 2006.

Streicher, Lauren F. *The Essential Guide to Hysterectomy.* M. Evans & Company, 2004.

HYSTEROSALPINGOGRAM

A hysterosalpingogram is an X-ray test that allows clinicians to see the inside of the uterus and fallopian tubes. The test is often done for women who are having a hard time becoming pregnant. More specifically, the test can be used to:

- Find a blocked fallopian tube, since infections can scar the fallopian tubes and prevent the passage of the eggs, thus preventing pregnancy.

- Find problems in the uterus, such as polyps, fibroids, adhesions, unusual shape, or other abnormalities. These conditions may cause miscarriages or painful menstruation.

- Discover whether surgery to reverse a tubal ligation has been successful.

HOW TO PREPARE
You should schedule your hysterosalpingogram for right after your period. Before you undergo a hysterosalpingogram, tell your doctor if you:

- Are pregnant or might be pregnant

- Have a pelvic infection or sexually transmitted disease

- Are allergic to iodine dye or any other substance that has iodine

- Have asthma or are allergic to any medications

- Have any bleeding problems or are taking blood-thinning medications

- Have a history of diabetes or kidney problems, especially if you take metformin for your diabetes (the dye used during a hysterosalpingogram can cause kidney damage in people who have kidney disease)

HOW IT IS DONE

A hysterosalpingogram is usually done by a radiologist at a clinic or hospital, possibly with the assistance of a radiology technologist, a nurse, and/or a gynecologist or reproductive endocrinologist. A few hours before the test, you may be asked to use a laxative or enema to empty the large intestine.

Before the test begins, you will be given a sedative or a mild pain killer (e.g., ibuprofen) and asked to lie on an examining table and put your feet in stirrups. A plain X-ray may be taken to ensure the large intestine does not contain anything that will block the view of the uterus and fallopian tubes.

The clinician will put a curved speculum into your vagina to allow him or her to see inside the vagina and the cervix. After the cervix is washed, a stiff or flexible tube will be put through the cervix into the uterus and the dye will pass through the tube. The clinician can follow the movement of the dye through the uterus and fallopian tubes on a monitor during the test. The entire test takes about fifteen to thirty minutes. Your doctor may request that you get another plain X-ray a few days after the procedure to make sure everything is fine.

BENEFITS

This test may uncover fibroids, polyps, scar tissue, or other abnormalities that may interfere with the ability to become pregnant. Occasionally the test flushes out blockages in the fallopian tubes, which then makes it easier to conceive.

RISKS/SIDE EFFECTS
Any exposure to radiation poses a potential risk to cells and tissue, but the level of radiation involved in this test is minimal and the benefits far outweigh the question of radiation. Other risks from a hysterosalpingogram include less than a 1 percent chance of a pelvic infection, endometritis, or salpingitis. Rarely, the uterus or fallopian tubes are punctured or damaged during the test. There is also a small chance of an allergic reaction to the iodine used in the X-ray dye or, if an oil-based dye is used instead, the oil can leak into the bloodstream and block blood flow to the lung.

After the procedure, do not have sexual intercourse or douche for at least two weeks.

READ MORE ABOUT IT
Ahmad G et al. Pain relief in hysterosalpingography. *Cochrane Database Syst Rev* 2007 Apr 18; (2):CD006106.

IN VITRO FERTILIZATION (IVF)

In vitro fertilization (IVF) is a technique that allows some infertile couples to produce a baby that is biologically related to them. Since IVF was first successful in 1981, more than 250,000 babies (sometimes known as "test tube babies") have been born using this approach.

Only about 5 percent of infertile couples use IVF, which is often the treatment chosen by women who have blocked, severely damaged, or no fallopian tubes. It is also helpful in women who are infertile because of endometriosis or because of problems with the man's sperm.

In vitro fertilization can involve the egg and sperm of the parents, or it may involve donated eggs, donated sperm, or donated embryos when one or both partners are unable to provide viable eggs or sperm.

HOW TO PREPARE

To prepare physically for in vitro fertilization, some doctors give their patients hormones (gonadotropins) to stimulate the ovaries to produce several eggs before the procedure to remove them is done.

Preparing emotionally for in vitro fertilization is critically important, as the process can be very stressful as well as expensive, placing both emotional and financial strains on couples. In vitro fertilization is a gamble: if the first cycle is not successful, then couples must decide if they will try again. It is important for couples who are considering IVF to seek guidance from fertility counselors and other trusted individuals.

HOW IT IS DONE

Using ultrasound as a guide, the surgeon inserts a needle through the vagina into the ovary to aspirate eggs. An alternative to this needle technique is laparoscopic surgery, but the needle approach is preferred. The fluid that is removed is examined to make sure there are eggs present. At the same time, the man provides a semen sample and the sperm are separated from the semen in a laboratory procedure. The eggs and active semen are then combined in a laboratory dish. Approximately eighteen hours later, it should be evident if one egg or several eggs have been fertilized and begun to grow as embryos.

The developing embryos are incubated and observed for two to three days or longer. The embryos are then transferred into the woman's uterus through the cervix using a catheter, with the hope that at least one will implant and develop naturally. The woman should stay in a resting position for an hour or two to facilitate the implantation. It is common to place two to four embryos in the uterus at one time to increase the odds of success. Each attempt is called a cycle.

For the next two weeks, the woman will take certain hormones. At the end of two weeks, she can take a pregnancy test to see if implantation was successful.

BENEFITS

One of the main benefits of IVF is that couples know before transfer takes place if the sperm has fertilized the eggs. If fertilization does not occur, changes can be made in how the semen is processed or in the fertilization conditions in the next attempt to create an embryo.

Another benefit is that the embryo is transferred to the uterus, which means the woman doesn't need to have functioning fallopian tubes for a pregnancy to occur.

RISKS/SIDE EFFECTS

A *New England Journal of Medicine* article reported that infants conceived by IVF have a 10 percent risk of birth defects, which is twice the risk of babies born naturally. Possible defects include holes in the heart, one kidney instead of two, cleft lips and palates, and brain abnormalities. Another study found that IVF children have a sixfold increased risk of having Beckwith-Wiedemann syndrome, a rare hereditary disorder that causes cancer.

Severe abnormalities in the eyes of IVF children also have been reported. Researchers found that because the children did not have a family history of the eye conditions found (e.g., glaucoma, cataracts), it was assumed that IVF was responsible.

READ MORE ABOUT IT

Riebeling P et al. Are screening examinations necessary in ruling out ocular malformations after reproduction treatment? *Klin Monatsbl Augenheilkd* 2007 May; 224(5): 417–21.

Sher, Geoffrey et al. *In Vitro Fertilization: The A.R.T. of Making Babies.* Facts on File, 2005.

INTRAUTERINE DEVICE (IUD)

An intrauterine device, or IUD, is a small, T-shaped device, that you can insert into your uterus to prevent pregnancy. When used correctly, the effectiveness rate of the IUD rivals that of the Pill: less than 1 percent of women get pregnant when using an IUD.

The IUD is unusual in that it must be inserted and removed by a health care professional, usually a physician or a nurse practitioner. Not all women are good candidates for an IUD; one should not be used by women who have any of the following conditions: pregnancy or suspected pregnancy, history of ectopic pregnancy, abnormal anatomy of the uterus, pelvic inflammatory disease or a history of the disease, any sexually transmitted disease, a positive test for HIV, fibroid tumors large enough to distort the uterus, a history of heavy menstrual bleeding and/or severe menstrual cramps, active cervical infection or an abnormal Pap test, any endometrial disorder (including endometriosis), heart disease, diabetes, liver disease, anemia, leukemia, clotting disorders, or current use of cortisone-type drugs or anticoagulants.

HOW TO PREPARE
Before getting an IUD, you should have a pelvic examination and review your history with your physician. Any tests to rule out infection and sexually transmitted diseases should be done if indicated.

HOW IT WORKS

Two types of IUDs are available in the United States, and both work in the same way: they prevent sperm from joining with an egg. One type contains copper and is effective for ten to twelve years; the other releases tiny amounts of progestin and is effective for five years. Copper is a material that helps prevent pregnancy, although experts are not completely certain how it works. Because copper causes inflammation of the endometrium, the theory is that the body responds to this inflammation by damaging sperm or by interfering with fertilization or implantation of the egg in the uterus. The progestin prevents the ovaries from releasing eggs, thus preventing pregnancy.

BENEFITS

Some of the benefits of using an IUD are:

- It is about 99 percent effective in preventing pregnancy.

- You don't need to interrupt sexual activity to insert a birth control device.

- The progestin-containing IUD often reduces the severity of cramps and the amount of bleeding during periods.

- You need to replace it just every five to ten years, depending on the type.

RISKS/SIDE EFFECTS

Most women adjust quickly to an IUD, but others may take weeks or months. The most common side effects associated with an IUD are spotting between periods, menstrual cramps, and backache. Over-the-counter pain relievers are usually effective. The copper type may cause a 50 to 75 percent increase in menstrual flow, which in turn may lead to a low red blood cell count. There is also an increased risk of pelvic inflammatory disease associated with IUD use.

Although serious problems with an IUD are rare, look out for these risks:

- An infection can develop if bacteria get into the uterus when the IUD is inserted. Most infections develop within three weeks of the insertion.

- An IUD can slip out of the uterus, either partly or completely. This is more likely to happen to young women who have never had a baby. If your IUD slips, your health care professional will need to reinsert it for you.

- Very rarely, an IUD is pushed through the wall of the uterus. In most cases the health care provider realizes this has occurred and can fix it immediately, but if it goes unnoticed (it usually is not painful), the IUD may move and injure other parts of the body. In these situations, surgery may be needed to remove the IUD.

READ MORE ABOUT IT
Fortney JA et al. Intrauterine devices. The optimal long-term contraceptive method? *J Reprod Med* 1999 Mar; 44(3): 269–74.

Kulier R et al. Copper containing, framed intra-uterine devices for contraception. *Cochrane Database Syst Rev* 2007 Oct 17; (4): CD005347.

KEGEL EXERCISES

Along with tummy crunches and butt tighteners, you need to strengthen your pelvic floor muscles, and Kegel exercises are just what you need to accomplish that. The pelvic floor muscles support your uterus, bowel, and bladder, three organs that can present some problems and discomfort if the supporting muscles become too lax.

Many things can weaken your pelvic floor muscles, including pregnancy, childbirth, chronic coughing, excess weight, getting older, and even a genetic predisposition for weak connective tissue in some women. When the pelvic floor muscles become weak, your pelvic organs "fall" and bulge into your vagina, a condition known as uterine prolapse. This condition can cause leakage of urine or feces and excess pressure in the pelvic region. One of the best ways to strengthen pelvic muscles is to practice Kegel exercises.

HOW IT IS DONE
It takes some patience and practice to do Kegel exercises correctly, but the benefits can be life-changing, especially if you are trying to prevent or control urinary or fecal incontinence. Follow these guidelines for doing Kegel exercises.

- To find your pelvic floor muscles, try to stop the flow of urine while you're going to the bathroom. If you succeed, you have found the right muscles and the basic action you need.

- If you were unable to stop the flow, insert a finger inside your vagina and try to squeeze the surrounding muscles. You should feel your vagina tighten and your pelvic floor muscles move upward. Relax your muscles, and you should feel your pelvic floor move down.

- Once you have identified your pelvic floor muscles, empty your bladder and either sit or stand comfortably. Tense your pelvic floor muscles for five seconds, then relax for five seconds. Repeat this sequence four to five times.

- Remember to breathe. Do not hold your breath while doing Kegel exercises.

- Do Kegel exercises at least three times a day, starting with five sets each time and gradually increasing to ten sets per session. The exercises will get easier the more you do them.

Note: do not do Kegel exercises when you have a full bladder or while emptying your bladder, because this can actually weaken the muscles and cause the bladder to not completely empty, which invites a urinary tract infection.

BENEFITS

Kegel exercises can strengthen pelvic muscles and delay or perhaps even prevent the prolapse of your pelvic organs. Some practitioners recommend that their pregnant patients practice Kegel exercises because well-toned pelvic muscles can make delivery easier and make women less likely to develop hemorrhoids and urinary incontinence, which are both common toward the end of pregnancy and postdelivery. Kegel exercises also may be helpful for women who have some difficulty reaching orgasm.

Allow about eight to twelve weeks before you'll see significant progress.

READ MORE ABOUT IT

Belo J et al. Pelvic floor muscle training with Plevnik's cones in women with urinary incontinence. *Acta Med Port* 2005 Mar–Apr; 18(2): 117–22.

ICON Health Publications. *Kegel Exercises: A Medical Dictionary, Bibliography, and Annotated Research Guide to Internet References.* ICON Health Publications, 2004.

Kielb SJ. Stress incontinence: alternatives to surgery. *Int J Fertil Womens Med* 2005 Jan–Feb; 50(1): 24–29.

MAMMOGRAPHY

Mammography is the use of low-dose X-rays to examine breasts to detect tumors and other changes in breast tissue. There are different types of mammograms:

- **Screening mammography** is used to detect breast changes in women who have no signs or symptoms of breast cancer. In most cases, two X-rays of each breast are taken.

- **Diagnostic mammography** is used to look for breast cancer after a lump or other sign or symptom of breast cancer has been detected. It is also used to evaluate changes found during screening mammography or to look at breast tissue that is difficult to evaluate because of factors such as breast implants. Diagnostic mammograms take longer than screening mammograms because they involve more X-rays and suspicious areas may be magnified to produce more detailed pictures.

- **Digital mammography** captures breast pictures digitally for viewing on a computer monitor, and the images are stored on a computer as compared with regular mammograms, which are stored on film in a cassette. Digital mammography allows clinicians to alter the magnification, orientation, contrast, and brightness of the images, which can help highlight certain areas. Some research indicates that digital mammography can expose women to up to 50 percent less radiation than conventional mammography.

HOW TO PREPARE

Make your appointment for one week after your period, because your breasts are least likely to be tender at that time. When you make the appointment, tell the office if you have breast implants. On your appointment day, do not use any perfume, antiperspirant, deodorant, lotion, or powder under your arms or on your breasts, because they can interfere with the quality of your mammogram.

HOW IT IS DONE

After you disrobe from the waist up, you will stand in front of an X-ray machine. The technician will place your breasts, one at a time, between two plastic plates, which come together to press your breast flat. You will feel pressure on your breast, which some women find mildly uncomfortable while others say it is painful. Each of the four X-rays—two pictures of each breast, one from the side and one from above—takes only a few seconds. A screening mammogram takes about fifteen minutes. A diagnostic mammogram, which involves more X-rays, takes about twice as long.

BENEFITS

Several large studies show that screening mammograms reduce the number of deaths from breast cancer for women ages forty to sixty-nine, and especially for those older than fifty. This benefit does not seem to extend to women younger than forty.

RISKS/SIDE EFFECTS

The only potential risk associated with getting mammograms is the exposure to radiation, which is minimal. There are no side effects. However, mammograms do have limitations. One is that it is only one part of a complete breast examination, so you should have your breasts examined by your physician or other qualified health care professional as well.

Another limitation is the possibility of a false negative, which means the mammogram looks normal but cancer is present. False negatives occur more often in younger women, who tend to have denser breast tissue than do older women. False positives—when mammogram results look like cancer is present but it is not—also are more common in younger women.

READ MORE ABOUT IT

Aydell, Carole. *Baring Your Breast: Mammograms: A Positive Experience.* AuthorHouse, 2008.

Berry DA. The screening mammography paradox: better when found, perhaps better not to find. *Br J Cancer* 2008 Jun 3; 98(11): 1729–30.

Berz D et al. "Weighing in" on screening mammography. *Breast Cancer Res Treat* 2008 May 20.

MASTECTOMY

A mastectomy is the surgical removal of the breast, usually as a treatment for breast cancer, although occasionally it is necessary in order to remove a very large benign growth. There are several kinds of mastectomy, and each one is defined by the amount of breast tissue and any other tissues that must be removed. The types of mastectomy most often performed today include radical, modified radical, simple (total), subcutaneous, and lumpectomy. (Some people argue that a lumpectomy should not be classified along with mastectomy, but it is increasingly grouped in that manner, so we have followed suit.) Each is described in more detail below under "How It Is Done."

In the past, women with breast cancer who were scheduled for a breast biopsy would allow the surgeon to decide whether or not the breast should be removed while they were anesthetized and so signed a consent form giving the doctor permission to do so. Today this is very rarely done, and the biopsy and ultimate surgery are done days if not weeks apart. This allows physicians more time to evaluate the biopsy and to decide if the tumor is hormone-dependent. It also gives you more time to decide which type of mastectomy you want and to choose a procedure that is based on more accurate and complete information than you would have if the surgeon proceeded directly from biopsy to mastectomy.

HOW TO PREPARE

Undergoing a mastectomy can cause a great deal of physical, emotional, and spiritual stress, and so it is important for you not only to attend to your medical needs but also to talk with or consult friends, family, or others who can support you emotionally and spiritually. Before the procedure, you may want to identify support groups or other resources you can turn to once the mastectomy has been done. In fact, you can attend mastectomy support groups before your procedure and talk with other women who have had a mastectomy so you can share your anxieties, fears, and questions.

Most mastectomy patients meet with their surgeon several days before the surgery to ask any questions and to sign a consent form. The anesthesiologist may also be present to talk about the plan for your anesthesia. You may also need to donate blood for a possible blood transfusion during surgery. Your surgeon will explain any presurgical preparations, such as refraining from any food or drink for at least eight hours before surgery.

HOW IT IS DONE

Mastectomy is usually done under general anesthesia with vital signs being monitored throughout the procedure, including heart rate monitoring with an electrocardiogram. The exact procedure depends on the type of mastectomy being done. For a simple mastectomy, for example, the surgeon makes an incision close to the tumor area and leaves most of the skin intact. The nipple is usually not removed, but the milk ducts leading to it are cut. The chest muscles and axillary (underarm) nodes are left intact. Sometimes the surgeon will do an axillary dissection of the lymph nodes nearest the breast to help determine how much, if any, the cancer has spread into the lymph nodes so postsurgery treatment can be decided.

The other four types of mastectomy include:

- **Radical mastectomy.** This procedure involves removal of the entire breast, nipple/areolar region, the major and minor chest muscles, and lymph nodes. It is rarely performed today except to treat advanced stages of breast cancer.

- **Modified radical mastectomy.** This is the most common type of mastectomy performed today. It involves removal of the entire breast and nipple/areolar region, and often the underarm lymph nodes.

- **Subcutaneous mastectomy.** This procedue involves removing the breast tissue only, sparing the skin, nipple, areola, chest wall muscles, and lymph nodes.

- **Lumpectomy.** This procedure involves the removal of the cancerous breast tissue and a surrounding rim of healthy breast tissue. A lumpectomy conserves the breast and is usually followed by radiation therapy to kill any residual cancer cells and as a precaution to help ensure the cancer does not return. Many surgeons also perform an axillary node dissection or sentinel node biopsy at the same time. This combination of procedures appears to yield survival rates that are as good as those with a total mastectomy.

Regardless of which type of surgical procedure you undergo, the surgeon will place a rubber or plastic drainage tube in the affected area to drain off excess fluids that will accumulate during the healing process. Drainage tubes are usually removed within fourteen days, or when the amount of drainage is less then 1 fluid ounce daily. The skin is closed with clips or stitches and a bandage is applied. A mastectomy with axillary lymph node dissection usually takes two to three hours. With axillary node dissection, usually ten to thirty lymph nodes are removed and examined in a lab to determine whether they contain cancer cells. A newer procedure, called a sentinel node biopsy, involves removing only the first one to three lymph nodes. If these nodes contain cancer, then additional surgery is needed to remove the remaining lymph nodes. If the first three lymph nodes are clear, then the cancer has not spread to the lymph system.

BENEFITS

Each type of mastectomy has its own benefits. A total mastectomy is aggressive, but it reduces the risk of the cancer spreading to other parts of the body. A modified radical mastectomy removes the chance of the cancer spreading to your lymph nodes, which could then spread (metastasize) to the brain or lungs. The benefit of a radical mastectomy is that it removes everything that could potentially spread to other parts of the body, and so it is similar to a total mastectomy. However, because a total mastectomy is less stressful and dangerous while providing the same results, radical mastectomies are rarely done. A subcutaneous mastectomy not only reduces the risk of spreading the cancer but also maintains the structure of the breast, which makes the job of the plastic surgeon easier if the woman wants to have breast reconstruction. A lumpectomy has survival rates similar to those of a total mastectomy, and so this less aggressive, less disfiguring approach is much preferred.

RISKS/SIDE EFFECTS

Possible risks or side effects associated with mastectomy depend on the type of mastectomy performed, although as with all surgical procedures there is a risk of infection. Other possible complications include:

- **Hematoma** (blood accumulation in the wound).

- **Seroma** (clear fluid trapped in the wound).

- **Numbness in the upper arm.**

- **Phantom breast pain.** This side effect affects about one-third of women who have had a mastectomy. The symptoms may include throbbing, pins and needles, unpleasant itching, and pressure. Massage and exercise may alleviate these symptoms, but in severe cases pan medication may be necessary.

- **Lymphedema** (if lymph nodes are removed). Up to 20 percent of women who have undergone mastectomy and axillary lymph node removal experience lymphedema, chronic swelling or tightness in the arm or hand caused by an accumulation of lymphatic fluid in the arm tissue. Approximately 400,000 breast cancer survivors live with this limitation every day.

- **Armpit vein thrombosis.** Women who have had axillary lymph node dissection are more prone to develop axillary vein thrombosis. That's because the unavoidable scarring that occurs because the lymph nodes were removed may narrow or kink the blood vessels and make them more susceptible to damage.

READ MORE ABOUT IT

Benedet, Rosalind. *After Mastectomy: Healing Physically and Emotionally.* Addicus Books, 2003.

Love, Susan M., et al. *Dr. Susan Love's Breast Book.* Perseus Pubishing, 2000.

Steligo, Kathy. *The Breast Reconstruction Guidebook.* 2nd ed. Carlo Press, 2005.

PAP SMEAR

The Pap smear (Papanicolaou test), also called a Pap test, checks for changes in the cervix, including infections, abnormal cells, or cervical cancer. Getting regular Pap tests is the best way for you to prevent cervical cancer, a disease that affects about 13,000 women per year in the United States and claims about 3,500 per year as well (see "Cervical Cancer").

The American Cancer Society recommends that women up to age thirty have a yearly Pap test. If you are thirty to sixty-five and have had three normal Pap tests for three years in a row, talk to your doctor about having a Pap test every two to three years. If you are sixty-five to seventy and have had at least three normal Pap tests and no abnormal Pap tests in the last ten years, talk to your doctor about stopping the tests.

HOW TO PREPARE

Getting a Pap test requires minimal preparation. Make your appointment for a time when you will not be menstruating, preferably ten to twenty days after the first day of your last period. Two days before your test, you should avoid douching, using tampons, or using any vaginal creams, suppositories, deodorant sprays or powders, or medications. It is also best to not have sexual intercourse within forty-eight hours of your test.

HOW IT IS DONE

A Pap test is done during a pelvic exam and takes only a few minutes. It is typically a painless procedure, but some women say it is uncomfortable. Much of the discomfort may come from stress and tensing your muscles, so it may be helpful to practice deep breathing or visualization to help you through it.

You will lie on an exam table and put your feet into stirrups. The doctor will put a speculum into your vagina, which opens up your vagina so your cervix can be viewed. A special swab or brush will be gently placed into your vagina and some sample cells taken from inside and around the cervix. The cells will be placed on a glass slide and sent to a laboratory for evaluation.

BENEFITS

Quite simply, a Pap test can save your life, because it can detect very early signs of cervical cancer, which allows you to get prompt treatment. Pap tests also can find infections and abnormal cervical cells that may develop into cancer cells.

RISKS/SIDE EFFECTS

There are no risks or side effects associated with having a Pap test. In fact, you are at risk if you do not have regular Pap tests.

READ MORE ABOUT IT

Palefsky, Joel, and Jody Handley. *What Your Doctor May* Not *Tell You About HPV and Abnormal Pap Smears.* Grand Central Publishing, 2002.

Rushing, Lynda, and Nancy Joste. *Abnormal Pap Smears: What Every Woman Needs to Know.* Prometheus Books, 2008.

PELVIC LAPAROSCOPY

Pelvic laparoscopy is a surgical procedure that examines and treats the pelvic organs (e.g., uterus, vagina, cervix, fallopian tubes, ovaries) through a small viewing instrument (laparoscope) that is inserted into the abdomen through a tiny incision near the navel. The procedure is used for both diagnosis and treatment. Your physician may recommend pelvic laparoscopy for any of the following reasons:

- Pelvic pain caused by endometriosis, pelvic inflammatory disease, an ovarian cyst, scar tissue in the pelvic area, or a twisted ovary

- A puncture of the uterus that occurred during a D&C or caused by an IUD

- Finding out why you are unable to get pregnant

- Removal of uterine fibroids

- Hysterectomy

- Surgical treatment of tubal pregnancy

Pelvic laparoscopy is not recommended if you are severely obese or if you have preexisting adhesions in the pelvic region.

HOW TO PREPARE

As soon as you know your surgery has been scheduled, tell your surgeon about any medications, herbs, and supplements you are taking. You will likely be asked to stop taking certain products, such as aspirin, for two weeks before surgery. You should not eat or drink anything after midnight before your surgery. You should also arrange for someone to drive you home after surgery.

If your physician believes there is a possibility that the laparoscope may not allow him or her to complete the needed surgery, you will be asked to sign a consent form stating that you give permission for your surgeon to do a full abdominal incision to complete the surgery.

HOW IT IS DONE

In most cases, pelvic laparoscopy is done under general anesthesia, but other anesthesias can be used that will allow you to stay awake. Once the anesthesia has taken hold, the surgeon will make a $1/2$-to-$3/4$-inch incision in the belly button or lower abdomen. Carbon dioxide gas is then passed into the abdominal cavity so the abdominal wall will move away from the organs, giving your doctor plenty of room to work.

A laparoscope (which contains a fiber-optic rod with a light and video camera) is then inserted through the incision. The video camera allows the surgeon to see inside the abdominal area on video monitors set up in the operating area. The surgeon then uses the video monitor as a guide as he or she performs surgery through the laparoscope by inserting specific instruments into the scope. If during the procedure your doctor discovers that surgery cannot be completed as necessary through the laparoscope, then a full abdominal incision will need to be made.

BENEFITS

The benefits of laparoscopy over conventional surgery are a short hospital stay (in the case of pelvic laparoscopy, you can usually go home the same day), faster recovery, minimal need for anesthesia, small scars, and mild to moderate postoperative pain.

RISKS/SIDE EFFECTS

The risks associated with a pelvic laparoscopy are similar to those with other surgical procedures, including infection, bleeding, and injury to nearby tissues and organs. Some people respond negatively to general anesthesia, including developing breathing problems.

After the procedure and during recovery, you may experience some abdominal discomfort for one to two days because of the carbon dioxide gas that is pumped into the abdomen for the surgery. Some women have some shoulder and neck pain for several days as the gas escapes through the skin. You can resume sexual activities as soon as any bleeding stops. If you have any persistent bleeding or fever or severe abdominal pain, you should call your doctor immediately.

READ MORE ABOUT IT

Katz, V. L., et al. *Katz: Comprehensive Gynecology.* 5th ed. Philadelphia: Mosby, 2007.

PESSARY

A vaginal pessary is a removable device that is placed into the vagina to support the pelvic organs. Pessaries are made of rubber, plastic, or silicone-based materials and come in several types, the most popular of which are the inflatable pessary, the doughnut, and the Gellhorn.

The most common use of pessaries is for treatment of pelvic organ prolapse (see "Prolapsed Bladder" in Part I). Although a pessary cannot cure prolapse, it can help manage and slow the progression of prolapse by supporting the vagina and increasing tightness of the muscles and tissues of the pelvis. For many women, wearing a pessary improves their symptoms, while for others it eliminates symptoms. Pessaries are frequently used in young women during pregnancy to treat uterine prolapse. They are also useful in women who have serious chronic health issues that make surgery too dangerous

HOW TO PREPARE

The only preparation necessary for wearing a pessary is getting properly fitted for one. A pessary is not a one-size-fits-all item: your physician or other health care professional will fit you for the device in the office. It often requires trying several different styles and sizes to find one that is not so loose that it comes out when you walk or strain or one that is not so tight that it causes abrasions.

HOW IT IS USED

Once you have been successfully fitted with a pessary, your health care professional will show you how to remove, clean, and reinsert it yourself, which should be done regularly, every six to eight weeks. If it is difficult for you to remove and reinsert your pessary, you can have it done regularly at your doctor's office.

BENEFITS

A pessary is an effective, noninvasive way to manage pelvic organ prolapse. Pessaries may be the best option if you are young and want to have children, if you have been told that surgery may be risky for you, or if you want to avoid surgery for your own reasons.

RISKS/SIDE EFFECTS

Wearing a pessary may cause some complications, including open sores in the vaginal wall, bleeding, irritation and erosion of the vaginal wall, and, in rare cases, bulging of the rectum against the vaginal wall, causing the formation of a rectocele. You can help prevent complications by cleaning your pessary frequently and having your health care professional check it if you feel the fit is wrong. If you are postmenopausal, use of estrogen cream or an estrogen ring may help eliminate irritation caused by the pessary.

If you have had a hysterectomy, you likely cannot wear a pessary because the uterus, which helps support the walls of the vagina, has been removed. You also cannot insert a diaphragm and wear a pessary at the same time. A pessary can be worn, without a diaphragm, during intercourse.

READ MORE ABOUT IT

Clemens JL et al. Patient satisfaction and changes in prolapse and urinary symptoms in women who were fitted successfully with a pessary for pelvic organ prolapse. *Am J Obstet Gynecol* 2004; 190(4): 1025–29.

Weber AM, Richter HE. Pelvic organ prolapse. *Obstet Gynecol* 2005; 106(3): 615–34.

TUBAL LIGATION

Tubal ligation, also known as "getting your tubes tied," is a surgical procedure that makes women sterile. The procedure involves either cutting, cauterizing, or blocking the fallopian tubes with rings, clips, or bands as a way to prevent eggs from traveling to the uterus from the ovaries. It also prevents sperm from reaching the fallopian tubes to fertilize an egg. The surgery is 99.5 percent effective as a birth control method, but it does not protect against sexually transmitted diseases. For women who have undergone tubal ligation and who then want to have the procedure reversed, there are surgeons who have had some success with reversal.

HOW TO PREPARE
When you sit down with your surgeon to discuss the surgery, tell him or her about any medications, herbs, or other supplements you are taking. You will probably be asked to stop taking certain medications, such as aspirin, for one to two weeks before the scheduled surgery. You should not eat or drink anything after the midnight before your surgery. If you are having same-day surgery, you should arrange to have someone drive you home after the procedure.

HOW IT IS DONE
In most cases, tubal ligation is an outpatient procedure that can be done in a clinic, doctor's office, or hospital, under either

local or general anesthesia. Some women choose to have their
tubes tied as part of a cesarean section or during childbirth.
When tubal ligation is not part of childbirth, most procedures
are done via laparoscopy (see "Pelvic Laparoscopy"). When
this method is used, the abdomen is filled with carbon dioxide
gas, which forces the abdominal wall to move away from the
internal organs, giving the surgeon room to work. The surgeon makes an incision just below the navel and inserts a
laparoscope, which has a light and a telescope-like instrument.
A second incision is made just above the pubic hairline, which
is where the instrument that will cut, burn, or sew the tubes
will be inserted. The entire process takes about thirty minutes.

After surgery, you should reduce your regular activities for
two to three days and wait at least one week, or until you feel
comfortable, before resuming sexual activity. If the procedure
was done through your vagina, you should avoid putting anything into your vagina for two weeks after surgery to avoid
developing an infection.

BENEFITS

Tubal ligation is considered to be a permanent form of birth
control (although it can be reversed in some cases) that is effective immediately after the procedure is over. Many women
report that they enjoy the freedoms that tubal ligation has offered them: they can be sexually spontaneous, there are no
pills or devices to deal with, and it is cost-effective in the long
run.

RISKS/SIDE EFFECTS

Possible side effects after tubal ligation include abnormal
bleeding and bladder infections. Although pregnancy is highly
unlikely, there is a slightly increased risk of ectopic pregnancy, which requires immediate medical attention. A condition called post-tubal-sterilization syndrome, which includes
irregular and painful periods, no periods, or midcycle bleeding, is reported by some women. Research into this syndrome
is being done.

READ MORE ABOUT IT

Gentile GP et al. Is there any evidence for a post-tubal sterilization syndrome? *Fertil Steril* 1999 Feb; 69(2): 179–86.

Peterson HB. Sterilization. *Obstet Gynecol* 2008 Jan; 111(1): 189–203.

ULTRASOUND

Ultrasound imaging, also called sonography, is a diagnostic tool that uses echoes of sound waves rather than radiation (X-rays) to provide an image of soft-tissue structures inside the body. The technology of ultrasound allows it to show the structure and movement of the internal organs and blood flow. Although it has many applications, ultrasound is especially useful in the diagnosis and treatment of women's reproductive and sexual health issues.

Conventional ultrasound can provide images in three or four dimensions, while Doppler ultrasound is a special technique that focuses on blood flow. Because ultrasound can make an outline of soft-tissue structures in a way that X-rays cannot, it is useful in monitoring a fetus and in detecting some defects. It can also distinguish between solid tumors and cysts of the ovaries and between some benign and malignant tumors. Clinicians often use ultrasound to guide needle biopsies and in amniocentesis (see "Amniocentesis" and "Biopsy"). A newer technique called high-definition imaging digital ultrasound is helpful in the detection of benign masses in the breast.

HOW TO PREPARE
Depending on the scan that is needed, you may be required to do nothing at all or be asked to abstain from food and liquids

for a period of time. If you are going to have an ultrasound of your baby and womb, you will likely be asked to drink four to six glasses of water about one to two hours before the examination. The extra fluid in the bladder moves the bowel away from the uterus so the technician can better view the baby and your womb during the ultrasound test.

HOW IT IS DONE

For most ultrasound sessions, you lie face up on an examination table that can be tilted. A clear gel is applied to the area to be examined. This allows the transducer (the device that both sends sound waves into the body and records the returning echo waves) to make firm contact with the skin. The ultrasound technologist or radiologist presses the transducer firmly against the skin and sweeps it back and forth over the area to be tested. In transvaginal ultrasound, the transducer is inserted into the vagina, which allows the clinician to view the uterus and ovaries. In most cases, ultrasound examinations take thirty to sixty minutes to complete.

BENEFITS

Ultrasound offers many advantages:

- Scanning does not involve needles or injections and is usually painless.

- It is widely available and less costly than other imaging techniques.

- It does not use radiation.

- It can provide pictures of soft tissues that are not clear on X-ray images.

- Because it is risk-free and painless, it can be repeated as often as medically needed.

- It provides real-time imaging, which makes it a reliable tool for guiding procedures such as needle biopsies and needle aspiration.

- It is a safe choice for pregnant women and their unborn children.

RISKS/SIDE EFFECTS
There are no known risks or side effects associated with ultrasound.

READ MORE ABOUT IT
Kanat-Pektas M et al. The evaluation of endometrial tumors by transvaginal and Doppler ultrasonography. *Arch Gynecol Obstet* 2007 Nov 29.

UTERINE FIBROID EMBOLIZATION

Uterine fibroid embolization is a minimally invasive procedure for treatment of fibroid tumors in the uterus (see "Fibroids" in Part I). This technique is used most often to treat
symptoms caused by fibroid tumors or to stop severe bleeding
caused by malignant gynecological tumors or childbirth. In
fact, the best candidates for this procedure are women who:

- Have fibroids that are painful or that are pressing on
  their bladder or rectum

- Have tumors that are causing significant bleeding

- Do not want to have a hysterectomy

- Already have children

HOW TO PREPARE
Tell your doctor about any medications and supplements you
are taking and if you have any allergies, especially to contrast
materials or anesthesia, and about any medical conditions,
including whether you are pregnant. Your doctor will likely
tell you to stop using aspirin or blood thinners for a week or
more before your procedure. The night before the procedure,
you should not eat or drink anything after midnight.

Once the fibroid tumors have been verified by magnetic

resonance imaging (MRI) or ultrasound, your physician may want to do a laparoscopy to get a direct look at the uterus. If bleeding is a major symptom, he or she may take a biopsy of the endometrium to rule out cancer.

HOW IT IS DONE

A uterine fibroid embolization is usually done by a specialist called an interventional radiologist. Once you are positioned on an examining table, you will be connected to monitors that track your heart, blood pressure, and pulse during the procedure. You will be given a sedative through an intravenous (IV) line and may also receive general anesthesia. A member of the surgical team will shave, sterilize, and cover the area of your body where a cathether will be inserted. The insertion site is numbed with a local anesthetic, and with the aid of X-ray guidance, a catheter is inserted through the skin into your femoral artery.

Contrast material may be sent through the IV to guide the catheter as the clinician guides it to your uterine arteries. Once the catheter reaches the fibroids, the embolic agent (substance that blocks blood flow) is injected until the blood flow in the uterine arteries that supply the fibroids is blocked. The catheter is then removed and the opening in the skin is covered with a dressing. No sutures are needed. The entire procedure takes about ninety minutes. In most cases, women stay in the hospital overnight so they can receive pain medication and be monitored.

BENEFITS

Uterine fibroid embolization is a good option for premenopausal women with symptoms of fibroid tumors who do not want to become pregnant and also do not want a hysterectomy. Unlike hysterectomy, which is commonly used to treat fibroids, uterine fibroid embolization is much less invasive, does not require a surgical incision, has a much faster recovery time, and does not require general anesthesia. The procedure is also an alternative for women who do not want to receive blood transfusions, which may be required during open surgery.

Research shows that approximately 85 percent of women who undergo uterine fibroid embolization have either significant reduction or complete elimination of their symptoms. On average, fibroids have shrunk to 50 percent of their original size six months after the procedure. Follow-up studies also show that fibroids treated with uterine fibroid embolization rarely grow back, unlike fibroids treated with hormone therapy or laser treatments.

RISKS/SIDE EFFECTS
The risks and side effects associated with uterine fibroid embolization are minimal and are far outweighed by the benefits, but they are worth noting.

- Anytime a catheter is placed there is a risk of damage to the blood vessel, bleeding or bruising at the puncture site, and infection. However, the chance of these events occurring is less than 1 percent when the procedure is done by an experienced interventional radiologist.

- Occasionally patients have an allergic reaction to the X-ray contrast material, which may range from mild itching to difficulty breathing. Because patients are monitored during the procedure, any allergic reactions can be immediately reversed.

- There is a slight chance that the embolic agent will lodge in the wrong place and deprive normal tissue of oxygen.

- One to 5 percent of women experience menopause shortly after undergoing uterine fibroid embolization. This occurs more often in women who are older than forty-five.

- Two to 3 percent of women may pass small pieces of fibroid tissue after the procedure. These women may need a dilatation and curettage (D&C; see "Dilatation and Curettage") to ensure all the tissue is gone so an infection will not develop.

- Less than 1 percent of women eventually need to have a hysterectomy because of infection or their symptoms persist.

- It is uncertain whether uterine fibroid embolization reduces fertility, so if you wish to become pregnant, you should talk to your doctor to discuss your options before having your fibroids removed with uterine fibroid embolization.

READ MORE ABOUT IT

McDaniel C. Uterine fibroid embolization: the less invasive alternative. *Nursing* 2007 Jul; 37(7): 26–27.

White AM, Spies JB. Uterine fibroid embolization. *Tech Vasc Interv Radiol* 2006 Mar; 9(1): 2–6.

MISCELLANEOUS TESTS

- **Alpha-fetoprotein (AFP) test.** A blood test used to check the level of AFP in a pregnant woman's blood. Levels of AFP indicate whether the infant may have such problems as omphalocele, spina bifida, or anencephaly. The AFP test can be done as part of a screening test to uncover Down syndrome and other chromosomal problems.

- **Amniography.** A type of X-ray procedure in which any structural defects in a fetus can be seen. It involves injecting a special dye into the amniotic sac and taking an X-ray, which with the dye more clearly shows the shape of the fetus. To avoid harming the fetus, this test is usually not done until late in pregnancy.

- **Estrogen-receptor assay.** A diagnostic test that can determine whether a cancerous tumor's growth depends on estrogen. Tumors that are estrogen-dependent typically do not respond well to chemotherapy, but they can respond to hormone manipulation, which can involve removing or inactivating organs and glands and/or taking large doses of hormones.

- **Nuchal translucency–biochemical blood test.** This test allows clinicians to test for fetal abnormalities very early in a pregnancy—between weeks 10 and 13. The test combines an ultrasound examination of the skin fold thickness at the back of the fetus's neck (which is greater in syndromes such as Down syndrome) with a measure of two biochemicals in the mother's blood that can signal possible chromosomal abnormalities. This test is used widely in Europe, where it can detect up to 90 percent of fetuses with Down syndrome. Although this test is not yet widely available in the United States, it is the subject of a government-funded study.

- **Percutaneous umbilical blood sampling.** This method can test for birth defects in the fetus's blood between weeks 18 and 36 of pregnancy. With the help of ultrasound, a needle is guided through the mother's abdomen and uterus into the umbilical vein, and the withdrawn blood is tested for most of the same conditions that can be detected using amniocentesis, but the results of this test are available in as few as twenty-four hours.

- **Radioreceptor assay.** This is an extremely sensitive pregnancy test that can give positive results in more than 99 percent of pregnant women before they miss a period. This blood test measures HCG (pregnancy hormone) at levels much lower than required by other pregnancy tests.

- **Rubin test.** Sometimes referred to as a carbon dioxide test, this procedure can detect obstructions in the fallopian tubes. The test can be conducted in an office or clinic and takes only a few minutes. Carbon dioxide gas is blown into the cervix and carefully monitored to see if the tubes are partly or wholly blocked. Sometimes the test itself unblocks a tube that had small bits of scar tissue or mucus. Because the test cannot reveal the nature of a tubal problem, clinicians typically use hysterosalpingography for fallopian tube obstruction.

- **Schiller test.** This diagnostic test for cervical or vaginal cancer involves coating the cervix and vagina with an iodine solution, which stains normal cells brown but is not absorbed by abnormal cells. If abnormal cells are found, clinicians usually order a colposcopy for further evaluation (see "Colposcopy").

- **Sentinel node biopsy.** A method for determining how far breast cancer has spread (also known as "staging"). It involves injecting radioactive and blue dyes at the tumor site and following their path. The first lymph node that receives drainage from a tumor is the sentinel lymph node. There can be more than one sentinel lymph node. If the node(s) do(es) not contain cancer cells, it is assumed that the remaining nodes also do not. This technique is just as reliable yet less invasive than standard lymph node dissection.

- **Sims-Huhner test.** Couples who are having problems with fertility may utilize this test, which determines whether a woman's cervical mucus is receptive to her partner's sperm. Within two to fifteen hours after a woman has had intercourse, she must visit her doctor or a clinic, where a sample of her cervical mucus is aspirated with a small suction catheter. If there are five or more actively moving sperm in the high-power field, the mucus is considered to be receptive enough for fertilization to occur.

MISCELLANEOUS INVASIVE PROCEDURES (SURGICAL AND NONSURGICAL)

- **Balloon ablation.** Also known as uterine balloon therapy, this is a method to relieve excessively heavy menstrual flow that is not caused by fibroids, cancer, or endometriosis. Balloon ablation is an outpatient procedure that involves inserting a balloon-tipped catheter through the vagina and cervix into the uterus. The balloon is filled with a sterile solution and a heating element heats the fluid until it reaches about 189°F. The balloon remains in place for about eight minutes, during which time the heat destroys the endometrial tissue. The balloon is then deflated, the fluid is drained, and the catheter removed.

- **Bilateral salpingo-oophorectomy.** The surgical removal of both ovaries and the fallopian tubes. It is indicated to treat cancer of the fallopian tubes, ovarian cancer, uterine cancer, and infected ovaries. This procedure is sometimes done at the same time as a hysterectomy.

- **Culdoscopy.** A procedure that involves inserting an instrument called a culdoscope through a small incision in the vagina, just behind the cervix, into the cul-de-sac. This allows a clinician to see the pelvic organs and determine whether the fallopian tubes are blocked or if there is an ectopic pregnancy. This technique is not used as much as it was in the past, and is often replaced by laparoscopy and mini-laparotomy.

- **Cystoscopy.** This procedure is performed by a urologist under local anesthesia and is used to diagnose interstitial cystitis. The examination involves inserting a slender instrument called a cystoscope through the urethra into the bladder. Samples of urine and tissue can be removed through the cystoscope for evaluation.

- **Embryoscopy.** A technique that allows clinicians to view a six-week-old embryo. It involves first inserting an ultrathin needle, which is guided by ultrasound, into the mother's abdomen. An endoscope attached to a camera is passed through the needle, which enables the clinician to see neural-tube and other defects.

- **Episiotomy.** A surgical incision made in the perineum (area between the vulva and the anus) during the second stage of labor to avoid tearing the perineal tissues. The incision is made in the bottom of the vagina when the baby's head is being delivered. If the mother has not been anesthetized, a local anesthetic is injected into the site where the incision will be made. After the baby is delivered, the incision is sutured.

- **Hysteroscopy.** A technique in which a visualizing instrument called a hysteroscope is inserted through the cervix into the uterus. With the help of a forceps attachment, it allows a physician to remove an IUD that has perforated the uterine wall. It can also be used to perform a tubal ligation or to remove uterine adhesions or fibroids. It requires local anesthetic and oral painkillers.

- **Hysterotomy.** A surgical procedure that goes through the uterine wall to terminate a pregnancy of 16 to 24 weeks. It is similar to a cesarean section in that the fetus and placenta are removed through a small incision. It is a risky procedure and should be reserved only for women who have medical problems that make other, safer methods impractical.

- **Mini-laparotomy.** A surgical procedure for tubal ligation that requires only local anesthesia and a one-inch incision. The clinician inserts a speculum into the vagina, clamps the cervix, and inserts an instrument called an elevator into the uterus. The surgeon makes a one-inch incision above the pubic bone and moves the elevator until the uterus is up against the incision. The fallopian tubes are located and then either cut, tied off, or cauterized. The surgeon then closes the incision with stitches. The woman can resume normal activities within a day or two.

- **Myomectomy.** A surgical procedure to remove fibroids. Rather than the more radical hysterectomy, which removes the entire uterus, a myomectomy involves removing the fibroid(s) only. The surgery is done under general anesthesia and can take from one to five hours.

- **Oophorectomy.** A surgical procedure to remove one or both ovaries. The former procedure is called unilateral oophorectomy; the latter is a bilateral oophorectomy. When both ovaries are removed, a woman is then sterile.

- **Salpingectomy.** The surgical removal of one or both fallopian tubes. This procedure is usually performed along with oophorectomy and/or hysterectomy.

- **Vaginoplasty.** A surgical procedure that tones the vaginal muscles and supportive tissues. Childbearing can significantly stretch the vaginal muscles, and a vaginoplasty can help you have greater contraction strength and control of your vaginal muscles. The procedure may also enhance your sexual experiences.

Q&A

Wasn't there some controversy about the safety of silicone gel breast implants? Are they safe?

Silicone gel breast implants first hit the market in 1962, and they were popular until the early 1990s, when there were safety concerns about a possible link between these implants and cancer, lupus, connective tissue disease, and the risk of ruptures. The implants were subsequently withdrawn from the U.S. market, and there was a flurry of independent studies that followed, for the purpose of deciding whether these implants were truly dangerous.

After more than a decade, the studies, including a report by the Institute of Medicine, found that silicone gel breast implants were not associated with these serious medical conditions. Thus the implants were reintroduced to the market in the United States on November 17, 2006. The Food and Drug Administration (FDA) approved them for breast enlargement for women age twenty-two years and older (the FDA says that a woman's breasts are not fully developed before that age). However, the two manufacturers of the implants must conduct postapproval studies, which will follow about 40,000 women for ten years after they receive their implants for indications of side effects and complications.

Therefore the long-term safety of silicone gel breast implants, which is still unknown, may be determined during this long-range observation period.

What is the success rate with in vitro fertilization?

Ten to 15 percent of women who undergo in vitro fertilization become pregnant on their first attempt with the procedure. Among this group of pregnant women, 25 percent will have a miscarriage. The success rate in achieving pregnancy is estimated to be no better than 30 percent with three attempts.

Can I have a vaginal birth if I had a cesarean section previously?

According to the American College of Obstetricians and Gynecologists, a vaginal birth after cesarean (VBAC) "is safer than repeat cesarean," and having had more than one previous cesarean does not pose any increased risk for women who want to have a vaginal birth. Of women who try VBAC, 60 to 80 percent are able to give birth vaginally. The success rate varies because it depends on why the previous birth was cesarean.

If you had a cesarean birth previously, it helps to know what type of incision you had. Cesarean births involve two incisions: one in the abdomen and another in the uterus. The type of incision in the uterus is not visible, but it is important for your doctor to know which type it is in order to avoid complications if you should elect to have a vaginal birth. Your medical records should state the type of incision that was made. If that information is not available, you may not be a candidate for VBAC.

There are three types of incisions: low transverse, low vertical, and high vertical. Women with high vertical incisions have a much greater risk of rupture of the uterus than women with another type of incision. Women who have had more than one previous cesarean delivery also may have an increased risk of rupture.

I want to have my tubes tied [tubal ligation] when I have my next (third) child delivered, and I'm wondering if it's 100 percent guaranteed that I'll never get pregnant again.

It is possible to become pregnant after you have had a tubal ligation, but the chances are pretty small: 2 to 10 women per 1,000 get pregnant after the procedure. If you did become pregnant, your pregnancy would most likely be normal, although there is a greater risk of ectopic pregnancy with a tubal ligation. Signs that you have a tubal pregnancy include pain and spotting after a missed period, a very light period, feeling dizzy or faint when pressure is placed on your bowels, and pain on one or both sides of the lower abdomen. If you experience any of these signs after you've had a tubal ligation, seek medical help as soon as possible.

What is the controversy about hysterectomies? How many of these procedures are unnecessary?

Some experts claim that only 10 percent of hysterectomies in the United States are necessary, and those are the ones performed for women who have cancer. However, among the remaining 90 percent of cases, there are likely many women who truly benefit from the surgery, even though they do not have cancer. These women typically elect to have a hysterectomy to treat severe pain and/or bleeding that has not responded to medication or other nonsurgical options.

Hysterectomy is the second most common major operation done in the United States, with approximately 600,000 women undergoing the surgery every year. The most common reason for doing the operation in the United States is to treat fibroids. The percentage of U.S. women who have had a hysterectomy is much greater than the percentage in other countries. For example, American women are twice as likely to have had a hysterectomy as women in England and four times more likely than Swedish women.

I've heard that an episiotomy can cause more problems than it solves. Is this true, and are there any alternatives?

The number of episiotomies has been declining in recent decades. Although the purpose of an episiotomy is to avoid tearing of the perineal tissue, researchers found that the procedure was causing more lacerations and complications than it was preventing. To avoid tearing the perineal tissue, some experts are recommending that women practice perineal massage, practiced daily for several weeks before delivery, and during labor as well. This massage seems to stretch the perineal tissue, although it cannot help the underlying muscle.

If I have breast implants, will I be able to breast-feed?

Most women who have breast implants who then want to breast-feed are able to do so. However, no reputable surgeon will guarantee that you will be able to breast-feed after breast augmentation or reconstructive surgery. The most surgeons can do is to promise to do their best. Several factors related to breast implant surgery can impact the ability to breast-feed after implantation. One is where the incision is made. A periareolar incision (near the areola) may disturb the ducts that carry milk from the breast lobe to the nipples. Another factor is where the implants are placed. Those positioned below the pectoral muscle usually have the least impact on the milk ducts. Thus you should discuss your plants to breast-feed when you consult with your plastic surgeon.

I am thirty-one years old and at very high risk of developing breast cancer. Both my sisters (one younger, one older) have been diagnosed with the disease, and our mother died of it. Should I have a preventive mastectomy?

This is a highly personal decision, and one that you should make with the guidance of qualified professionals, including genetic and psychological counselors who can discuss the psychosocial impacts of the surgery and what to expect after surgery. You may also want to discuss your decision with your loved ones. We also recommend that you get a second opinion.

You certainly have one of the main risk factors for considering this preventive surgery: a family history of multiple cases of breast cancer, especially those diagnosed before age fifty. Other factors that place women at high risk of developing breast cancer are a personal history of previous breast cancer, presence of breast-cancer-causing genes (e.g., BRCA1 or BRCA2), and presence of lobular carcinoma in situ, a condition that increases the risk of developing breast cancer.

Preventive mastectomy involves removing one or both breasts in order to prevent or reduce the risk of breast cancer. One of two basic procedures can be done: a total mastectomy or a subcutaneous mastectomy (see "Mastectomy"). Most doctors recommend a total mastectomy because it removes more tissue than a subcutaneous procedure, thus providing you with more protection against cancer.

Preventive mastectomy may reduce the risk of developing breast cancer in moderate- and high-risk women by about 90 percent. When it comes to how satisfied women are who had preventive mastectomy, a National Cancer Institute study found that of 519 women who had preventive mastectomy, 86.5 percent were satisfied with the procedure and had no second thoughts about it and 76 percent were very content with their quality of life.

No procedure can completely eliminate your chances of getting cancer. Just because you cut away a breast, cancer can still develop in the area where the breast used to be. Preventive mastectomy is a choice, and you should take advantage of any information you can gather plus the advice of professionals and loved ones in making your final decision.

Is there any reason why a mother should not breast-feed?

The decision to breast-feed is a personal one, and one that a woman should discuss with her obstetrician. Before we answer your question about why you may not be able to breast-feed, let's mention some of the benefits. For infants, breast milk is the most complete form of nutrition, far better than anything you can buy off the shelf. Not only does mother's milk contain the right amount of protein, water, sugar, and fat necessary for your baby's growth and development, it is also easier to digest than formula.

Breast-fed babies get antibodies from mother's milk, and these substances protect infants from viruses and bacteria, making them less likely to get infectious diseases including ear infections, diarrhea, respiratory illnesses, and other conditions. Breast-fed infants are less likely to be hospitalized, require fewer doctor's visits, and have lower rates of diabetes, lymphoma, leukemia, obesity, high cholesterol, asthma, and sudden infant death syndrome (SIDS).

Breast-fed infants tend to be a little leaner than formula-fed babies and also less likely to become overweight later in life. Breast-fed babies also score higher on IQ tests.

As a breast-feeding mom, you can benefit because nursing uses up calories, which makes it easier to lose extra pounds from the pregnancy. Nursing also helps the uterus return to its original size and delays the return of normal ovulation and your period. Studies show that breast-feeding reduces the risk of developing breast and ovarian cancers later in life.

Breastfeeding is a bargain: you don't need to buy formula and spend the time to measure and mix it and then warm up bottles. "Dinner is always ready," says Melissa, a thirty-one-year-old first-time mom. "When I'm too tired to get up, I don't have to. I just put a nipple into her mouth and the café is open for business!" And perhaps the most priceless benefit is that breast-feeding is the ultimate in bonding time between mother and child. Physical contact is critically important for infants, and breast-feeding mothers also experience greater feelings of closeness and self-confidence because they have breast-fed.

Medically, there are very few reasons why a woman would be advised not to breast-feed. One is if you are receiving long-term chemotherapy; another is if you have human immunodeficiency virus (HIV). If you are taking medications that can be transferred into breast milk (as many drugs can) and those drugs can harm your baby, you can talk to your doctor about possible safe substitutions for those drugs or stopping the drugs temporarily while you breast-feed. If these options are not feasible for you, then you may not be able to breast-feed.

I am thinking about starting hormone replacement therapy, but I'm interested in bioidentical hormones. Where can I get them? Do I need a prescription?

Bioidentical hormones are substances that have the exact same molecular structure as the hormones that your body makes, and so they cause your body to react in the same way as it would to the body's natural hormones. The Food and Drug Administration, which oversees drugs and drug manufacturing in the United States, considers bioidentical hormones, which are derived from plants, to be natural and so they, like herbal products such as garlic tablets or dandelion tea, cannot be patented. Synthetic hormones are patented, and their manufacturers do not like the competition from bioidenticals.

Bioidentical hormones are prescribed by a physician and are available in two ways: FDA-approved preparations that have been formulated with strict oversight and are dispensed by pharmacies; and those compounded by a licensed pharmacist who knows how to prepare customized hormone preparations. To find a compounding pharmacy near you, visit the following Web site: www.angelfire.com/fl/endohystnhrt/pharmacy .html, where pharmacies are listed by state.

There are some genetic problems in my family and I'd like to have an amniocentesis. I'm ten weeks pregnant now. How soon can I have the test? How long will it take for me to get the results?

A genetic amniocentesis, which is usually given to women who are 35 years or older who have an increased risk of chromosomal abnormalities, is usually done after the fifteenth week of pregnancy. It can accurately identify certain genetic disorders, such as Down syndrome and spina bifida, but it can't identify heart defects, cleft lip, cleft palate, or clubfoot. A maturity amniocentesis, which is done to determine if the baby's lungs are mature enough, is done after the thirty-sixth week of pregnancy.

Lab results take various amounts of time. For genetic analysis, some results may be ready after just a few days, but traditional chromosomal evaluations can take up to fourteen days, which is how long is necessary for the fetal cells to multiply sufficiently so there are enough to be tested. Results of maturity amniocentesis are available within hours.

PART III

Getting What You Need: Quality Health Care

The health needs and concerns of women change continuously, and this is especially true when it comes to both physical and emotional issues associated with reproductive and sexual health. From amenorrhea and breast cysts to menopause and uterine fibroids, dozens of conditions are largely hormone-driven. Sometimes we may feel that these surging chemicals in our bodies have taken over. But there are other factors contributing to our health challenges as well, and understanding how all these factors come together to make us who we are can be a daunting task.

Today most women want to take control of and responsibility for their own health, and one way to do that is to seek information from reliable sources from the media and from qualified professionals in the conventional and complementary realms. In the previous two sections of this book we brought you the latest information on reproductive and sexual health conditions and some ways they can be prevented and treated. In this section we offer you guidelines on how to enhance the knowledge you are gaining about your health: how to find the right health care professionals to partner with you on your health care. Whether you are looking for a gynecologist, an obstetrician, a midwife, or a genetic counselor, we provide guidelines and checklists to help you make your selection. We also offer important information that may serve to enhance your understanding and appreciation of various reproductive and sexual health concerns, including birth control options and reliability, cancer staging, and a look at chemotherapy options for breast, cervical, ovarian, and endometrial cancers.

HOW TO FIND THE RIGHT
HEALTH CARE PROFESSIONAL

Part of taking control of your own health care involves finding and have a relationship with the right health care professionals. If you are reading this section, you are probably in
the market for some professional guidance. In the realms of
reproductive and sexual health, there are many specialists
who can be instrumental in your getting the care you need
and deserve. We look at several of those specialists and offer guidelines on how to find the right one for your unique
needs.

FINDING A GYNECOLOGIST
Your relationship with your gynecologist can be a special
one, especially if you have some very specific reproductive, ·
menopausal, postmenopausal, and/or sexual issues. Some
women are happy to depend on their family physician, inter-
nist, or nurse practitioner for routine gynecological exams
and screenings and turn to a specialist (gynecologist and/or
obstetrician) if other concerns arise. Others prefer to see their
gynecologist for everything related to reproductive and sexual health, from routine screenings to minor procedures and
testing, even surgery in some cases. As forty-one-year-old
Pamela puts it, "I treat my body better than I treat my car. If I
had a Mercedes, I'd bring it to a discount oil change place,
though I'd go to a Mercedes dealer for more significant work.
But my body gets top-notch care from the start. I want a

doctor who is familiar with my basic history of Pap smears, breast exams, and so on, if I should ever need something serious or more complicated attended to. So I go to a gynecologist that I carefully chose for all my women's health needs."

So how do you go about choosing a gynecologist? (Although some gynecologists are obstetricians as well, we look at how to choose an obstetrician as a separate issue below.) It takes a little planning, but it is time well spent. Many women ask their female friends and family members for recommendations, which is certainly one thing you can consider. However, you and your friends may not see eye to eye on selections, so you should take some time to search further. Before you begin, you can save yourself some time and energy if you decide at the beginning whether you prefer a male or female gynecologist. Once you have decided, here are some suggestions to help you with your search:

- **Identify your needs.** Do you need a gynecologist who practices general gynecology or one who may specialize in, say, endometriosis or cervical cancer? Do you want a gynecologist who is also an obstetrician? Do you want someone who understands any specific cultural or social beliefs or needs you may have? Do you need a doctor who is close to where you live because of transportation issues? Do you need a gynecologist who speaks a language other than English?

- **Check with your insurance carrier.** Some plans allow you to choose your own gynecologist in addition to a primary care provider; others require you to use a gynecologist from a list that your primary care physician refers you to.

- **Choose a gynecologist who is board-certified in obstetrics and gynecology.** This is different from a board-eligible physician, which means a doctor who has met the requirements to take the board exam but has not yet taken it. A board-certified doctor has full credentials—has completed an accredited four-year residency training program, done a specified number of surgical procedures after residency, and passed the accrediting obstetrics and gynecology board exams.

- **Consult with other physicians, especially women.** Women physicians and nurses can be great resources for information, especially if they have personal experience with a gynecologist in your area. If they recommend someone, ask what makes this doctor so special for them.

- **Contact your county medical society.** They can give you the names of physicians in your area who may meet your needs. Remember, however, that such societies cannot endorse or recommend physicians.

- **Call the doctor's office.** Note how your call is handled. Was it difficult to get through to a live person? Was the receptionist polite? If the receptionist was unable to answer your questions, did she or he refer you to someone who could, or were your questions basically ignored? Some questions you might ask on that initial call are: How long much patients typically wait past their scheduled appointment time? If the doctor must leave for an emergency (typical of obstetricians), how are the appointments scheduled for that time handled—does an associate take over? Does the doctor have weekend and/or evening hours? How long does it take to get an appointment? Does the doctor reserve special times for routine examinations and other times for problem-related visits?

- **Ask for an initial interview with the doctor.** This is a getting-to-know-you visit, so that you will know if you feel comfortable with this physician. Here are some topics you may want to discuss during your visit:

- What are the doctor's thoughts about alternative medicine?

- Does the doctor prescribe natural hormones?

- If you are planning on having a baby, what are the doctor's approaches to labor and delivery?

- If you are approaching menopause, how does the doctor feel about hormone therapy or herbal therapy?

- How are after-hours medical emergencies handled?

- If the doctor is unavailable, will you be passed along to an associate?

- Is the doctor open to receiving phone calls with questions, or is e-mail an option?

- How long has the doctor been in practice?

- Which hospitals is the doctor associated with?

During your getting-to-know-you visit, you should also note how the doctor responds to you. Does the doctor encourage you to ask questions, or do you sense impatience or condescension? Does the doctor ask you questions and seem truly interested in you and your concerns? Overall, how does the doctor make you feel? Go with your gut feeling here. Although gut feelings are not "scientific," they are often the most important barometer of how the relationship will proceed.

FINDING AN OBSTETRICIAN
Many of the questions you would use to find a gynecologist you can also use to find the right obstetrician, so we did not bother to repeat them here—simply refer to "How To Find the Right Gynecologist" above. However, there are some very spe-

cial concerns and questions you need to address when looking for an obstetrician or obstetrician/gynecologist. So here are some guidelines to consider.

- Is the doctor certified by the American College of Obstetricians and Gynecologists?

- How many babies has the doctor delivered?

- Will the doctor help you with your birth plan?

- Which hospitals and/or birth centers is the obstetrician affiliated with?

- Does the doctor's practice use interns or residents? Some women are comfortable with up-and-coming doctors being involved in their pregnancy and delivery; others are not.

- Who provides backup if the obstetrician cannot attend the birth?

- What percentage of the obstetrician's fees will be covered by your insurance?

- What is the obstetrician's recommended schedule of prenatal visits? What is the typical length of time of each visit?

- How does the obstetrician feel about including a midwife in your delivery?

- Under what circumstances would the obstetrician induce labor?

- What tests does the obstetrician typically order during pregnancy?

- What type of support does the doctor provide for breast-feeding?

- What percentage of the doctor's deliveries are cesarean? Induced labor? If either of these numbers is high, you will want to know why. High numbers may, but not necessarily, indicate that the doctor does these procedures for his or her convenience.

- How does the doctor feel about natural childbirth?

- How much time will the obstetrician spend with you while you're in labor?

- What are the obstetrician's views on offering pain relief during labor and/or delivery?

FINDING A CERTIFIED NURSE-MIDWIFE

Certified nurse-midwives (CNMs) are individuals who have been trained in both nursing and midwifery and are certified by the American College of Nurse-Midwives (ACNM). Certified nurse-midwives are licensed to practice in all 50 states and can provide a wide range of services to women, including routine gynecological checkups, preconception care, prenatal and postpartum care, and delivering babies. They will attend a birth wherever it takes place, whether it's a hospital, birth center, or private home. Another classification of midwives are direct-entry midwifes, who usually do home births. They may be certified by the North American Registry of Midwives, and their legal status varies among the states.

Why Choose a Midwife?

Some women want a more individualized, personalized, and less routine approach to pregnancy and childbirth, and midwives can offer these benefits. Some women say their midwife is like their best girlfriend who helps them through the physical and emotional ups and downs of pregnancy while also offering professional advice on diet and how to make pregnancy and the birthing experience memorable events.

Certified nurse-midwives are there to help and support your birth plan. If you want any tests that the CNM cannot do herself (e.g., amniocentesis, ultrasound), then she will make the arrangements for you. If a medical or obstetrical condition arises, such as gestational diabetes or multiple birth, that requires the attention of an obstetrician or a perinatalogist (a doctor who handles high-risk pregnancies), she will refer you to one. If you initially choose a nonmedicated labor and you decide at the last moment you want an epidural during labor, CNMs have obstetricians available for consultation and backup if needed.

Who Can Use a Midwife?

If you are in good health, which means you do not have any chronic condition such as diabetes, high blood pressure, or heart disease, then you can likely engage the services of a midwife. Studies show that healthy women with normal pregnancies who choose CNMs were just as likely as those who choose an obstetrician/gynecologist to have excellent outcomes with childbirth. Women who choose certified nurse-midwives also tend to have fewer medical interventions, such as epidurals, continuous electronic fetal monitoring, and episiotomies. They also have a lower rate of cesarean sections.

Choosing a Certified Nurse-Midwife

You should choose your midwife as carefully as you would an obstetrician and/or gynecologist. That means you will have an initial getting-to-know-you visit so you can ask questions and see if you are comfortable with the midwife. Here are some questions you could ask during your visit.

- How long have you been in practice?

- Where do you practice most often—hospital, homes, birthing centers?

- How many babies have you delivered?

- How many babies do you typically deliver in one month?

- Did you graduate from a nationally accredited midwifery education program? If so, which one?

- Are you certified by the American College of Nurse-Midwives?

- Are you licensed by the state?

- How much time do you spend during each prenatal visit?

- What is the average waiting time in your office?

- How can I reach you if there is an emergency?

- Which obstetricians do you work with?

- Who covers for you if you are not available?

- If you are in a group practice, how often will I see the other practitioners? Do they share your same philosophy?

- Do you have hospital admitting privileges? If yes, which hospital?

- Which prenatal tests do you typically recommend?

- Under what circumstances might you manage my care jointly with a doctor or transfer my care to a doctor?

- Will you help me develop a birth plan?

- Will you stay with me throughout labor?

- What do you suggest for pain during labor?

- What percentage of your patients have episiotomies?

- What percentage of your patients have a cesarean?

- If I need a cesarean, will you stay with me throughout the procedure?

- How long will I be separated from my baby after the birth?

- May my baby room with me?

- Will you or one of your staff help me with breast-feeding?

- Questions to ask yourself about the midwife:

  - Did she make you feel comfortable?

  - Did she encourage you to ask questions and seem genuinely interested in you and your needs?

  - If your partner went with you, did the midwife include both of you in the conversation?

  - How long did you have to wait past your appointment time?

  - Is the support staff friendly and helpful?

FINDING AN INFERTILITY SPECIALIST: REPRODUCTIVE ENDOCRINOLOGIST

If you are reading this section, you probably strongly suspect or you have been told by a health care professional that you and/or your partner are infertile. Infertility is defined as the inability to conceive after one year of unprotected intercourse or, if you are thirty-five years or older, after six months of unprotected intercourse. If you fit into either of these categories, or if you have had two spontaneous miscarriages, you should see an infertility specialist.

An infertility specialist is an ob-gyn (obstetrician/gynecologist) who has been specially trained in reproduction and infertility issues. An ob-gyn is trained to diagnose and treat general disorders and diseases of the female reproductive system and to provide care during pregnancy, childbirth, and postpartum. Some ob-gyns have some knowledge of infertility, but they have not been specially trained in advanced reproductive methods.

Infertility specialists—or more accurately, reproductive endocrinologists—represent a subspecialty of ob-gyn that focuses on treating infertility for both women and men. Thus reproductive endocrinologists are board-certified by the American Board of Medical Specialties after having completed a two-to-three-year fellowship in infertility treatment, followed by two years of clinical experience. They must also pass oral and written exams. All of this special training is above and beyond the four-year ob-gyn residency training and board certification. These are very highly trained individuals.

A highly trained individual does not necessarily translate into someone you are comfortable with, however. It is critical that you have a good rapport with whomever you choose, because you will be sharing some very intimate information with this professional. Thus an initial getting-to-know-you appointment is important. If possible, schedule an appointment with more than one reproductive endocrinologist.

Interviewing a Reproductive Endocrinologist
Both you and your partner should go to the interview session. Go with a prepared list of questions. The ones provided here are a good starting point:

- Where did you receive your medical training? How long have you been in practice as a reproductive endocrinologist?

- Are you board-certified as a reproductive endocrinologist?

- If you are unable to see me, do you have other reproductive endocrinologists on staff?

- Whom can I call if I have a problem after office hours?

- Do you answer e-mails from patients?

- Are you affiliated with a hospital, and if so, which one?

- Are you a member of the American Society for Reproductive Medicine?

- How much does treatment cost?

- Which insurance plans do you accept?

- Do you accept payment plans or financing options?

- Do you have a donor sperm or donor egg program?

Your Initial Assessment

Once you've made your selection and it's time for you to schedule your appointment for your assessment, try to make it during the first week of your menstrual cycle. If you have been recording your basal body temperature and/or your ovulation cycle, bring this information with you to your appointment. The specialist will ask you many questions about your sex life as well as about your current health, menstrual history, pregnancy history, types of birth control you have used, any history of sexually transmitted infections, family health history, dietary habits, amount of exercise, and whether you use any drugs (alcohol and nicotine included), legal or illegal.

The doctor will do a physical exam and check your thyroid

and do both a breast and pelvic examination. A sample of cervical mucus may be collected for evaluation, and blood tests will probably be ordered to measure your hormone levels. If other problems are suspected, such as polycystic ovary syndrome, a vaginal ultrasound may be ordered.

Once a diagnosis has been made, treatment can begin. For many couples, "low-tech" solutions are found; for example, going to couples therapy, use of fertility drugs, or treating an underlying condition such as pelvic inflammatory disease. A small percentage of patients seek help with assisted reproductive methods, such as in vitro fertilization (see "In Vitro Fertilization" in Part II).

In Vitro Fertilization Clinics

If in vitro fertilization (IVF) is your treatment choice, you will need to select an IVF clinic. There are approximately 375 IVF clinics in the United States. The average success rate for assisted reproductive methods is about 28 percent, which is 50 percent higher than unassisted conception. However, not all clinics have similar success rates, nor do they all offer the same procedures or services, and fees vary considerably as well.

When choosing an IVF clinic, be sure it is accredited by the College of American Pathologists, the Joint Commission on the Accreditation of Healthcare Organizations, or the state. The clinic should also follow the guidelines established by the American Society for Reproductive Medicine and preferably be a member of the Society for Assisted Reproductive Technology, an indication that the clinic and staff are keeping current with technology.

Here are some questions to consider when choosing an IVF clinic:

- What procedures do you offer? Are they all offered on site?

- How many board-certified reproductive endocrinologists are on staff?

- Do you have a laboratory on site?

- Does the clinic offer counseling?

- Is the clinic affiliated with a hospital, and if yes, which one?

- What is the cost of treatment, including lab work and drugs?

- What insurance plans do you accept?

- Are donor sperm or donor eggs available?

- Is the clinic open on weekends?

- Do you offer patient education programs?

FINDING A PLASTIC SURGEON
A plastic surgeon is called in to do breast augmentation or reconstruction. If you are undergoing a mastectomy, your surgeon may be able to recommend a plastic surgeon or two for you to consider. If possible, it is best to select your plastic surgeon before you have the mastectomy so the two surgeons can consult on your case and help you better prepare for the reconstruction. Here are some suggestion to help you with your search:

- **Check board certification.** Look for a physician who has been certified by the American Board of Plastic Surgery (ABPS), which is the only board recognized by the American Board of Medical Specialties to certify doctors in plastic surgery.

- **Check membership.** Check to see if your plastic surgeon is a member in good standing with the American Society of Plastic Surgeons (ASPS) and/or the American Society for Aesthetic Plastic Surgery (ASAPS).

- **Check facility accreditation.** Make sure the facility where the surgery is done is accredited. Some cosmetic surgery is done in office-based surgical facilities, and many of them are not accredited. ASPS and/or ASAPS member surgeons operate only in accredited facilities.

- **Check hospital privileges.** Make sure the surgeon has operating privileges in an accredited hospital for the procedure you are considering.

CANCER STAGING

Your doctor has told you that you have cancer and that it's at stage III. What does this mean? We're confident that your doctor will explain it to you, but it's also good to have a place you can turn to for basic information.

The stage of a cancer reflects the degree to which it has progressed. Knowing the stage of your cancer determines what type of treatment your doctor will pursue with you and also gives some clues about the chances of cure and potential life expectancy. Thus accurate staging is critically important. If you have any questions about the staging of your cancer, talk to your physician.

Below is a brief overview of staging for breast, ovarian, and uterine (endometrial) cancer. See the Appendix for resources for more information on cancer.

BREAST CANCER STAGING

- **Stage I.** The tumor is less than 2 cm in diameter with minor skin involvement. It may or may not be attached to the chest wall, muscle, or fascia. The axillary nodes have no evidence of cancer, and there is no evidence of metastasis.

- **Stage II.** The tumor is between 2 cm and 5 cm and it may be attached to the chest wall or muscle. Movable axillary nodes contain cancer, and there is no evidence of distant metastasis. This stage can also refer to a larger tumor if there is no axillary node involvement.

• **Stage IIIA.** The tumor is larger than 5 cm with or without attachment or extension to the chest wall or fascia. The axillary nodes contain cancer and are attached to each other or to other structures. There is no evidence of distant metastasis.

• **Stage IIIB.** The tumor can be any size with metastasis to skin, the chest wall, or internal mammary lymph nodes.

• **Stage IV.** The tumor can be any size and has extension to the skin or chest wall. The supraclavicular (above the clavicle [collarbone] at the base of the neck) or infraclavicular (below the clavicle) nodes contain cancer, or the arm has edema. There is also evidence of distant metastasis.

ENDOMETRIAL CANCER STAGING

• **Stage 0.** The tissue sample is suspicious but nothing can be proven.

• **Stage I.** Cancer is confined to the body of the uterus.

• **Stage IA.** Cancer involves less than half of the myometrium.

• **Stage IB.** Cancer involves more than half of the myometrium.

• **Stage II.** Cancer is located in both the uterus and cervix.

• **Stage III.** Cancer has extended outside the uterus but not outside the pelvis.

• **Stage IV.** Cancer has extended outside the pelvis or has involved the mucosa of the rectum or bladder.

OVARIAN CANCER STAGING

• **Stage I.** Cancer is limited to the ovaries.

  • **Stage IA.** Cancer affects one ovary only, and there is no ascites (accumulation of serous fluid).

  • **Stage IB.** Cancer affects both ovaries and there is no ascites, although there is serous fluid in the peritoneal cavity.

  • **Stage IC.** Cancer affects one or both ovaries and ascites is present with malignant cells in the fluid.

• **Stage II.** Cancer affects one or both ovaries with extension to the pelvis.

  • **Stage IIA.** Cancer affects one or both ovaries, with extension and metastasis to the uterus and fallopian tubes.

  • **Stage IIB.** Cancer affects one or both ovaries, with extension and metastasis to other pelvic tissues.

• **Stage III.** Cancer involves one or both ovaries, with widespread metastasis to the abdomen.

• **Stage IV.** Cancer involves one or both ovaries with distant metastasis outside the peritoneal cavity.

SCREENING GUIDELINES FOR EARLY DETECTION OF CANCER IN ASYMPTOMATIC WOMEN
(American Cancer Society)

- **Pap test (for cervical cancer).** All women who are or have been sexually active or have reached age eighteen should have an annual Pap test and pelvic exam (see "Pap Test" in Part II).

- **Pelvic examination.** From ages eighteen to forty, women should have a pelvic exam every one to three years; after age forty, every year.

- **Endometrial tissue sample.** Taken at menopause and thereafter if your doctor suspects you are at high risk.

- **Breast self-examination.** All women age twenty and older should do a self-exam every month.

- **Breast examination, clinical.** Women ages twenty to forty should have one every three years; after age forty, every year.

- **Mammography.** Women forty to forty-nine, every one to two years; women fifty and older, every year.

- **Fecal occult blood test (for bowel cancer).** Women older than fifty should have one yearly; it can be done as part of the annual pelvic examination.

- **Digital rectal examination.** Women older than forty should have one done every year; it can be a part of the annual pelvic examination.

EFFECTIVENESS OF BIRTH CONTROL METHODS

Method	Effectiveness (Estimated)
Abortion	100%
Cervical cap w/spermicide	
Women with children	60–74%
Women without children	80–91%
Condom (Male)	86–97%
Diaphragm w/spermicide	80–94%
Hysterectomy	100%
IUD	
Copper	99%
Progesterone	98.5%
Oral contraceptives	95–99.5%
Spermicide alone	
(foam, jelly, suppository)	74–93%
Tubal ligation	99.5%

CHEMOTHERAPY DRUGS

If you should need to take chemotherapy drugs, talk to your doctor about all the pros and cons, side effects, expected results, and other questions you may have. The following list of chemotherapy drugs is representative of those often used by women who have reproductive cancers.

- **Doxorubicin (Adriamycin).** This drug belongs to the class of anthracyclines, and it is both a type of antibiotic and an anticancer drug that helps to slow or stop the growth of cancer cells in the body. It is given intravenously to treat various conditions, including breast, cervical, and endometrial cancers. Doxorubicin can cause a decline in the number of blood cells in your bone marrow, which lowers your resistance to infection. Prolonged use of this drug is associated with severe heart damage, even years after you stop taking the drug. Other side effects caused by doxorubicin include nausea and vomiting, diarrhea, difficulty swallowing, thinned hair, skin irritation or rash, hand-and-foot syndrome (swelling, pain, redness, or peeling of skin on the palms and soles of the feet), and loss of appetite.

- **Cisplatin (Platinol-AQ).** This drug is given intravenously to treat metastatic ovarian cancer and cervical cancer. Use of cisplatin can cause a decrease in the number of blood cells in your bone marrow, which can significantly compromise your immune system. It can also cause a severe form of kidney impairment and hearing loss. Other common side effects include diarrhea, nausea and vomiting, thinning hair, tingling in the hands and feet, loss of appetite, and changes in taste.

- **Cyclophosphamide (Cytoxan).** In a drug class called alkylating agents, cyclophosphamide slows or stops the growth of cancer cells. It is given either intravenously or orally to treat breast and ovarian cancers. The most common side effects include nausea, vomiting, and irritation of the urinary bladder.

- **Methotrexate (Folex, Mexate, Amethopterin).** This drug is classified as an antimetabolite, which means it interferes with the metabolism of cells, including cancer cells. It is given intravenously and is associated with some very serious side effects, including life-threatening damage to the lungs, kidneys, bone marrow, and lungs. It should not be used during pregnancy or lactation, as it can harm the baby.

- **Fluorouracil (5-FU).** This anticancer drug is given intravenously to treat breast and ovarian cancers, among other conditions. More than 30 percent of people who take 5-FU experience diarrhea, mouth sores, nausea and vomiting, poor appetite, and low blood counts.

- **Taxanes; paclitaxel (Taxol, Abraxane), docetaxel (Taxotere).** The classification taxanes includes drugs used to treat breast, ovarian, and endometrial cancers. Taxol has been approved for early and advanced breast cancer, Taxotere for locally advanced or metastatic breast cancer, and Abraxane for advanced or recurrent breast cancer. These drugs are associated with common side effects, including anemia, low platelet count, low white blood cell count, cough or hoarseness accompanied by chills or fever, flushed face, lower back or side pain, painful or difficult urination, shortness of breath, rash, and itching.

- **Epirubicin (Ellence).** This drug is in a class called anthracyclines and is given intravenously for treatment of breast cancer. It can cause severe heart damage, even months to years after taking it. It can also lower blood cell levels and has been associated with the development of new cancers.

- **Capecitabine (Xeloda).** This drug converts to 5-FU in the body and is used to treat metastatic breast cancer. Capecitabine is given orally and can cause lymphopenia (low white blood cell levels, which compromises the immune system) in nearly all patients who take it. It is also associated with a very high occurrence of anemia, nausea and vomiting, severe diarrhea, hand-and-foot syndrome, and fatigue.

- **Gemcitabine (Gemzar).** This anticancer drug is classified as an antimetabolite and is used to treat metastatic breast cancer. It is given intravenously. Side effects experienced by 30 percent or more of patients who take the drug include flulike symptoms, fever, fatigue, nausea and vomiting, poor appetite, rash, and low blood counts, which increases your risk for infection, bleeding, and/or anemia.

- **Vinorelbine (Navelbine).** This drug is given intravenously or orally for advanced breast cancer. Nearly all patients experience a significant decline in various types of white blood cells, which can severely compromise the immune system. Vinorelbine is also associated with a high risk of anemia, nausea, vomiting, constipation, and peripheral neuropathy.

It is common practice to combine anticancer drugs as part of a patient's chemotherapy treatment plan. Here are some often-used cancer drug combinations and their acronyms, which are used extensively by health care professionals.

- CMF: cyclophosphamide, methotrexate, and fluorouracil

- CAF (or FAC): cyclophosphamide, doxorubicin, and fluorouracil

- AC: doxorubicin and cyclophosphamide

- EC: epirubicin and cyclophosphamide

- TAC: docetaxel, doxorubicin, and cyclophosphamide

- AC to T: doxorubicin and cyclophosphamide followed by paclitaxel or docetaxel

- A to CMF: doxorubicin followed by CMF

- A CEF: cyclophosphamide, epirubicin, and fluorouracil (with or without docetaxel)

- TC: docetaxel and cyclophosphamide

- GT: gemcitabine and paclitaxel

A CLOSER LOOK AT BREAST LUMPS

A breast lump is a growth that may have distinct borders, or it may feel like a general thickened mass of tissue in the breast. In most cases, breast lumps are benign, although occasionally they are a sign of breast cancer (see "Breast Cancer" in Part I). That's why your doctor should promptly evaluate any lump you may find in your breast. Some of the more common causes of breast lumps include breast cysts, fibroadenomas, and fibrocystic breast changes, all of which are covered in detail in Part I. Other less common causes of breast lumps are explained below.

- **Fat necrosis.** A painless, firm, round lump most often found in obese women who have very large breasts. The lump typically forms in response to trauma, such as a blow to the breast, even though the woman may not remember the incident.

- **Galactocele.** A cystic tumor that contains milk and is formed when a duct becomes obstructed during lactation. Galactoceles typically develop at the end of breast-feeding when the milk stagnates in the breast ducts, although often the lump is not discovered until months later. Galactoceles usually can be treated by aspirating the milk with a needle.

- **Hamartoma.** An uncommon benign tumorlike growth that consists of disorganized cells and tissues normally found in the area where the growth occurs. Usually hamartomas are composed of fat, glandular tissue, and fibrous connective tissue. Most are seen in women older than thirty-five years and do not cause any symptoms. A biopsy is usually needed to make a diagnosis.

- **Intraductal papilloma.** This is typically a small, benign tumor that grows in a milk duct in the breast near the nipple. Intraductal papillomas are the most common cause of spontaneous discharge from the nipple from a single duct. You or your health care professional may feel a small lump beneath the nipple, but intraductal papillomas cannot always be felt. Mammograms often do not show papillomas, but ultrasound may reveal it. A bruise or bump near the nipple can cause the papilloma to bleed. Single intraductal papillomas are more common in women as they near menopause, while multiple papillomas are more common in younger women. Multiple intraductal papillomas often develop in both breasts. Most experts recommend that any intraductal papilloma that is associated with a lump be removed.

- **Lipoma.** A lipoma is a slow-growing, fatty tumor that usually is not painful or tender. It has a distinctive way of moving readily when slight finger pressure is applied, and it is doughy to the touch. These growths are usually harmless and don't require treatment unless they become painful or grow too large, in which case they can be removed.

- **Phyllodes tumor.** Similar to a fibroadenoma (see "Fibroadenoma" in Part I), a phyllodes tumor develops from the lobules in the breast. They are rare and can be cancerous and metastasize. Phyllodes tumors vary greatly in size but may grow to encompass the entire breast, at which point it is necessary to remove the breast.

- **Sclerosing adenosis.** This benign, often painful lump is the result of excessive growth of tissues in the lobules of the breast. Sclerosing adenosis is usually difficult to distinguish from cancer, so biopsy is usually necessary to make the diagnosis.

GLOSSARY

Adenocarcinoma: A cancer that develops in the lining or inner surface of an organ.

Adhesion: A thick layer of connective tissue that forms over a healing cut, abrasion, or other type of lesion. When adhesions form in the fallopian tubes, cervix, or uterus, they can cause infertility.

Amenorrhea: Failure to menstruate at an age when regular menstruation is normal, in the absence of pregnancy or breast-feeding.

Amniotic sac: Sometimes referred to as the "bag of waters," it is a membrane that develops around a fertilized egg about one week after fertilization and eventually surrounds the fetus. It has many functions, some of which are protecting the fetus against possible injury, maintaining an even temperature, and serving as a fluid source for the fetus.

Androgens: Male hormones that promote the development of male sexual characteristics. Testosterone is the main androgen.

Areola: The ring of brownish or pink skin that surrounds the nipple of the breast.

Axillary: Referring to the armpit or under the arm.

Benign: Describes a tumor or other growth that is not cancerous.

Birth plan: A plan for the birthing process that includes the woman's or couple's wishes (e.g., use of pain medication, involvement of a midwife, type of delivery) as well as allowances for special circumstances and complications or emergency situations.

Board-certified: A designation given after a physician passes a difficult examination and receives certification by an official medical specialty board. The American Board of Medical Specialties recognizes twenty-four specialty boards and also some subspecialties. Board certification does not guarantee outstanding care, but it does verify that a physician who claims to be a surgeon, for example, is really a surgeon.

CA-125: A protein that acts as a cancer marker (indicator). It is normally made by certain cells, including those of the uterus, the cervix, and the lining of the abdomen and chest. It is measured in a blood sample.

Cervicitis: Inflammation of the cervix, usually caused by infection but occasionally by chemicals or a foreign body (e.g., IUD, tampon).

Clitoris: A cylindrical structure at the upper front of the vulva, located just above and in front of the urethral opening. It is usually less than 1 inch long, even when erect, and its only known function is for sexual pleasure.

Clomiphene citrate: A drug used as part of infertility treatment to stimulate the release of hormones needed to initiate ovulation. Typically it is taken for five consecutive days early in the menstrual cycle for three to six monthly cycles. It can take several cycles to find the right dose. Once the dose is determined, a woman will

take the drug for at least three more cycles unless she is successful in getting pregnant. If pregnancy does not occur after six cycles, it usually means clomiphene treatment will not be successful.

Clue cells: Cells in the vagina that are covered with bacteria,
uniquely found in women who have a vaginal infection.

Complicated abortion: Any spontaneous or induced abortion
that results in complications, such as bleeding or infection.

Cone biopsy: Also called conization, it is the surgical removal of a
cone-shaped piece of tissue from the cervix. It is done to determine whether cancerous cells are present.

Contraceptive sponge: A soft, disposable polyurethane object
that serves as a birth control method. It measures about 2 inches
around, fits over the cervix, and is preloaded with spermicide.
Once inserted into the vagina, it traps and kills sperm and blocks
the cervix.

Corpus luteum: The structure that forms after the follicle bursts
and releases the egg. The purpose of the corpus luteum is to produce progesterone until the placenta can take over production,
which occurs at approximately ten weeks' gestation.

Cystitis: A type of urinary tract infection; inflammation of the
bladder.

Cystocele: A condition in which the bladder bulges into the vaginal canal. It often occurs along with prolapsed uterus and is usually the result of childbirth.

Dilatation and curettage (D&C): A technique used mainly for
induced abortion and to remove endometrial polyps.

Dilatation and evacuation: A surgical procedure and abortion
method in which the cervix is dilated and the contents of the

uterus are removed (evacuated). It is normally performed during the second trimester.

Douching: Rinsing the vagina with water or another solution, including vinegar and water, yogurt, and herbal teas. Most experts agree that douching is rarely necessary and encourages rather than eliminates vaginal infections because it upsets the acidity of the vagina and the bacterial balance.

Dyspareunia: Painful sexual intercourse.

Dysuria: Painful or difficult urination.

Ectopic pregnancy: A pregnancy in which the fertilized egg implants outside the uterus, usually within a fallopian tube, and begins to develop there.

Endometrium: The lining of the uterus, which thickens in response to hormonal changes each month and then sloughs off during the menstrual cycle.

Endovaginal ultrasound: A painless imaging test that allows clinicians to examine the pelvic organs. Endovaginal ultrasound (also called transvaginal ultrasound) is best for diagnosing ovarian cysts, and it provides good images of the pelvic organs (e.g., uterus, ovaries, fallopian tubes, cervix, vagina).

Episiotomy: A surgical procedure in which an incision is made in the bottom of the vagina as the baby's head is being delivered.

Estrogen replacement therapy: The use of either natural or synthetic estrogen, taken orally, by injection, as a cream or suppository, or in a patch, primarily to relieve symptoms of menopause.

Fallopian tubes: The two narrow passages, located on either side of the uterus, which transport eggs from the ovaries.

Fibroid: A noncancerous growth, ranging in size from a pea to a large grapefruit, that occurs in about 20 percent of all women older than thirty-five.

Follicle-stimulating hormone: A hormone produced by the pituitary gland that is involved in regulating the activity of the sex glands. Follicle-stimulating hormone (FSH) works along with luteinizing hormone (LH) to stimulate the development of the graafian follicle, a sac that contains eggs in the ovary.

Gamma-linolenic acid (GLA): An essential polyunsaturated fatty acid found in some plant seed oils including evening primrose oil, black currant oil, and borage oil.

High-risk pregnancy: A general term used for pregnancy in women who have a chronic disease or another condition that makes pregnancy high-risk for them and/or their babies. Examples of such chronic conditions include heart disease, diabetes, liver disease, alcoholism, AIDS, and high blood pressure.

Hot flashes: A sudden sensation of heat that usually begins in the chest and passes up to the neck and face, typically causing the latter two areas to become sweaty and flushed. This reaction may be followed by excessive perspiration and chills. Hot flashes can last from several seconds to several minutes and recur many times an hour or as little as once or twice a year.

Hymen: A thin elastic membrane that partly covers the vaginal opening, allowing menstrual blood to flow out. Although some cultures consider the tearing or stretching of the hymen to indicate that a girl/woman has had sexual intercourse, the hymen can be compromised by activities such as horseback riding, gymnastics, or ballet, or by use of tampons or insertion of fingers into the vagina.

Induced abortion: The intentional termination of a pregnancy, using drugs or surgical methods, before the fetus reaches the stage where it can survive outside the body.

Infertility: The inability to conceive after twelve months of regular, unprotected (without birth control) sexual intercourse or, in women thirty-five years and older, after six months of unprotected sex.

In vitro fertilization (IVF): A procedure in which a number of eggs are removed from a woman's ovaries after they have been stimulated by a fertility drug, and then are fertilized by a man's sperm in a laboratory. Children born as a result of IVF are sometimes known as "test tube babies."

Intrauterine device (IUD): A device composed of plastic, metal, or other material that is inserted into the uterus to prevent pregnancy. It must be inserted and removed by a trained health care practitioner and can stay in place for five to ten years, depending on the type of IUD used.

Kegel exercises: Exercises designed to strengthen the muscles of the pelvic floor in order to prevent urinary incontinence, strengthen orgasmic response, and prepare for and recover from childbirth. They are also known as pelvic floor exercises.

Labia: The two sets of tissue folds that protect the vaginal opening. The outer, larger pair of labia (labia majora) are composed mainly of fatty tissue. The inner pair of labia (labia minor) are two flat, firm, reddish folds that extend down from the clitoris.

Lactobacilli: Lactobacilli is a genus of bacteria that has many species, perhaps the most well known of which is *L. acidophilus,* that are involved in keeping the gastrointestinal tract healthy. *L. acidophilus* and other lactobacilli species are found naturally in the body and can also be taken as supplements called probiotics.

Libido: The desire to engage in sexual activity; also known as sex drive.

Luteinizing hormone (LH): A hormone released by the pituitary gland that controls the length and sequence of the menstrual cycle, production of estrogen and progesterone by the ovaries, and preparation of the uterus for implantation of a fertilized egg.

Lymph nodes: Small, bean-shaped structures of tissue that are located along the vessels of the lymphatic system, which is a critical part of the immune system. Lymph nodes are essential because they filter bacteria and cancer cells from the lymphatic fluid.

Lymphedema: A common, chronic condition in which fluid called lymph accumulates in the tissues, causing swelling (edema), especially in the arms and legs.

Malignant: A term used to describe a tumor or growth that is cancerous.

Mastectomy: A term used generally to describe the surgical removal of the breast, but it also encompasses lumpectomy, which is the removal of only the tumor and a small amount of surrounding breast tissue. The main types of mastectomy are radical, modified radical, simple, lumpectomy, and subcutaneous.

Mastitis: An inflammation of the breast usually caused by the bacteria *Staphylococcus aureus,* but occasionally by other organisms. It is usually contracted during breast-feeding.

Masturbation: The practice of sexually stimulating oneself to orgasm.

Menstrual cycle: The regular, roughly monthly process of preparing the lining of the uterus for the implantation and support of a fertilized egg; if no egg is fertilized, it ends in the shedding of the lining (menstruation). This cycle is regulated by the fluctuations and interactions of various hormones.

Metastasis: The spread of disease, usually cancer, from one part of the body to another that is not directly connected to it.

Midwife: An individual other than a physician who is trained to assist during childbirth. Although there are lay midwives, who often do not have formal training, nurse-midwives are registered nurses who have taken special postgraduate training in gynecology and obstetrics to be qualified to care for women before, during, and after childbirth.

Mini-laparotomy: A type of abdominal tubal ligation in which the incision is very small and only local anesthesia is needed.

Minipill: A form of oral contraception (the pill) that contains only a small dose of progestin and no estrogen.

Miscarriage: The loss of a pregnancy or expulsion of a fetus before it has developed sufficiently to survive outside the mother's body. It is also called a spontaneous abortion or natural abortion.

Myometrium: The muscular outer layer of the uterus.

Neural tube defects: A group of common, very serious birth defects that involve the failure of an infant's spinal cord to close properly. When the failure is at the top of the spine, the condition is called anencephaly, a condition that is usually fatal within hours of birth. When the failure is lower on the spinal cord, the condition is called spina bifida.

Obstetrician: A physician who specializes in obstetrics, which includes childbirth, prenatal care, delivery, and postpartum care.

Oophorectomy: The surgical removal of one or both ovaries. Also called ovariectomy.

Ovulation: The regular release of an egg (or ovum) from the ovaries, which roughly occurs monthly except during pregnancy, beginning soon after menstrual periods start (menarche) until after menopause.

Perimenopause: The two to six years or so that precede the end of menstruation. It is characterized by irregular menstrual periods and mood swings, loss of concentration, and hot flashes.

Perineal massage: A technique that involves slowly and gently stretching the tissues around the vagina and perineum in an effort to ease the passage of an infant during childbirth and reduce the risk of tearing the skin and the need for an episiotomy.

Placenta: The organ that connects a fetus to its mother and allows the exchange of oxygen, nutrients, and secretions. The placenta is connected to the fetus by the umbilical cord.

Polyp: A fleshy, noncancerous tumor that is usually attached to normal tissue by a stem. Polyps found in the female reproductive system include cervical and endometrial polyps.

Postpartum: The first six weeks after childbirth.

Prevalence: The number of cases of a disease that exists in a given population at a specific time.

Probiotics: A term referring to dietary supplements and/or foods that contain beneficial or "good" bacteria that are similar to those that occur naturally in the body. Beneficial bacteria provide many health benefits, such as providing protection against disease-causing bacteria and aiding digestion.

Progestin: Synthetic or "look-alike" progesterone, called medroxyprogesterone. The chemical structure of medroxyprogesterone resembles that of natural progesterone, but the differences can result in different responses.

Prolactin: A hormone that is released by the pituitary gland and that stimulates breast development and milk production in women.

Rectocele: A bulging of the wall of the rectum into the vagina. It may occur alone or along with a prolapsed uterus and/or cystocele.

Screening: The examination of individuals (usually symptom-free) to detect if there are signs of a specific disease.

Serous fluid: Any of various body fluids resembling serum, especially lymph.

Signs: An objective indication of a disorder or disease, such as swelling, bleeding, or fever, which can be seen and/or measured by a clinician.

Sitz bath: Also known as a hip bath, it is a type of bath in which only the hips and buttocks are soaked in water. It is used to ease the pain of uterine cramps, ovaries, hemorrhoids, inflammatory bowel disease, and vaginal and bladder infections.

Spontaneous abortion: A miscarriage; an abortion that was not artificially induced.

Squamous cell carcinoma: A type of cancer that begins in squamous cells (thin, flat cells that look like fish scales). Squamous cells are found in the tissue that forms the lining of hollow organs (e.g., vagina, uterus).

Symptom: Subjective evidence of a disorder or disease, which the patient can feel or is experiencing but which cannot be seen by the clinician. Examples include pain, dizziness, and fatigue.

Tamoxifen: An antiestrogen drug (a drug that blocks the effects of the hormone estrogen) that is used to treat breast cancer and help prevent the disease in women who are at high risk for the disease.

Thyroid-stimulating hormone (TSH): A hormone produced by the pituitary gland that promotes the growth of the thyroid gland

and stimulates it to produce more thyroid hormones. When thyroid hormones reach high levels, the pituitary gland stops producing TSH, which reduces thyroid hormone production.

Urethra: In women, the narrow tube that lies in front of the lower part of the vagina. The urethra carries urine from the bladder to outside the body.

Urethritis: An infection or inflammation of the urethra. This is a common disorder that often occurs along with a bladder infection, or it may be associated with gonorrhea, trichomoniasis, chlamydia, or other infections of the vagina.

Vaginal cancer: A rare form of cancer typically seen only in women whose mothers were treated with diethylstilbestrol during their pregnancy.

Yeast infection: One of the most common vaginal infections, it is caused by a yeastlike fungus called *Candida albicans.*

APPENDIX

Sources of online and print information, support groups, forums, videos, research articles, and much more.

ALTERNATIVE MEDICINE FOUNDATION
www.amfoundation.org
PO Box 60016
Potomac, MD 20859
301-340-1960

AMERICAN ASSOCIATION OF BIRTH CENTERS
www.birthcenters.org
3123 Gottschall Road
Perkiomenville, PA 18074
215-234-8068

AMERICAN ASSOCIATION OF SEX EDUCATORS,
COUNSELORS AND THERAPISTS
www.aasect.org
PO Box 1960
Ashland, VA 23005-1960
804-752-0026

AMERICAN COLLEGE OF NURSE-MIDWIVES
www.midwife.org
8403 Colesville Road, Suite 1550
Silver Spring, MD 20910
240-485-1800

AMERICAN SOCIAL HEALTH ASSOCIATION
www.ashastd.org
PO Box 13827
Research Triangle Park, NC 27709
800-227-8922 (STD Information Hotline)

AMERICAN SOCIETY FOR AESTHETIC PLASTIC SURGERY
www.surgery.org
11081 Winners Circle
Los Alamitos, CA 90720-2813
888-272-7711

AMERICAN SOCIETY FOR COLPOSCOPY AND CERVICAL PATHOLOGY
www.asccp.org
152 W. Washington Street
Hagerstown, MD 21740
800-787-7227

AMERICAN SOCIETY FOR REPRODUCTIVE MEDICINE
www.asrm.org
1209 Montgomery Highway
Birmingham, AL 35216-2809
205-978-5000

AMERICAN SOCIETY OF PLASTIC SURGEONS
www.plasticsurgery.org
444 E. Algonquin Road
Arlington Heights, IL 60005
847-228-9900

AMERICAN UROGYNECOLOGIC SOCIETY
www.augs.org
2025 M Street, NW, Suite 800
Washington, DC 20036
202-367-1167

BREAST CANCER ALLIANCE
www.breastcanceralliance.org
15 E. Putnam Avenue, Number 414
Greenwich, CT 06830
203-861-0014

BREAST CANCER NETWORK OF STRENGTH
www.networkofstrength.org
212 W. Van Buren Street, Suite 1000
Chicago, IL 60607-3903
800-221-2141

ENDOMETRIOSIS ASSOCIATION
www.endometriosisassn.org
8585 N. 76th Place
Milwaukee, WI 53223
414-355-2200

GILDA RADNER FAMILIAL OVARIAN CANCER REGISTRY
www.ovariancancer.com
Roswell Park Cancer Institute
Elm and Carlton Streets
Buffalo, NY 14263-0001
800-682-7426

HERPES RESOURCE CENTER
www.herpesresourcecenter.com
2990 Panorama Drive
N. Vancouver, BC, Canada V7G 2A4

HERS FOUNDATION
www.hersfoundation.org
422 Bryn Mawr Avenue
Bala Cynwyd, PA 19004
610-667-7757
888-750-4377

INTERNATIONAL POF ASSOCIATION
www.pofsupport.org
PO Box 23643
Alexandria, VA 22304
703-913-4787 (Support Line)

INTERNATIONAL SOCIETY FOR THE STUDY OF VULVOVAGINAL DISEASE
www.issvd.org
8814 Peppergrass Lane
Waxhaw, NC 28173
704-814-9493

LA LECHE LEAGUE INTERNATIONAL
www.llli.org
PO Box 4079
Schaumburg, IL 60168-4079
877-4-LALECHE (Breast-feeding Helpline)
847-519-7730 (Leader Locator)

MIDWIVES ALLIANCE OF NORTH AMERICA
www.mana.org
611 Pennsylvania Avenue, SE, #1700
Washington, DC 20003-4303
888-923-6262

NATIONAL ABORTION FEDERATION
www.prochoice.org
1660 L Street, NW, Suite 450
Washington, DC 20036
202-667-5881

NATIONAL ASSOCIATION FOR CONTINENCE
www.nafc.org
PO Box 1019
Charleston, SC 29402-1019
800-252-3337

NATIONAL CANCER INSTITUTE
www.cancer.gov/cancertopics/types/breast
6116 Executive Boulevard, Room 3036A
Bethesda, MD 20892-8322
800-422-6237

NATIONAL CERVICAL CANCER COALITION
www.nccc-online.org
6520 Platt Avenue, Number 693
West Hills, CA 91307
800-685-5531

NATIONAL UROLOGICAL ASSOCIATION FOUNDATION
www.UrologyHealth.org
1000 Corporate Boulevard
Linthicum, MD 21090
866-746-4282

NATIONAL VULVODYNIA ASSOCIATION
www.nva.org
PO Box 4491
Silver Spring, MD 20914-4491
301-299-0775

PLANNED PARENTHOOD FEDERATION OF AMERICA
www.plannedparenthood.org
434 West 33rd Street
New York, NY 10001
212-541-7800

POLYCYSTIC OVARIAN SYNDROME ASSOCIATION
www.pcosupport.org
PO Box 3403
Englewood, CO 80111

PREECLAMPSIA FOUNDATION
www.preeclampsia.org
5353 Wayzata Boulevard, Suite 207
Minneapolis, MN 55416
800-665-9341

RESOLVE: THE NATIONAL INFERTILITY ASSOCIATION
www.resolve.org
1760 Old Meadow Road, Suite 500
McLean, VA 22102
703-556-7172

**SHARE: SELF-HELP FOR WOMEN WITH BREAST
OR OVARIAN CANCER**
www.sharecancersupport.org
1501 Broadway, Suite 704A
New York, NY 10036
212-719-0364

VULVAR PAIN FOUNDATION
www.vulvarpainfoundation.org
PO Drawer 177
Graham, NC 27753
336-226-0704

HOTLINES

American Institute of Ultrasound in Medicine:
800-638-5352

Female Health Foundation (STDs, birth control):
800-635-0844

Genetic Alliance (genetic counseling):
800-336-4363

Hysterectomy Educational Resources and Services:
888-750-HERS

Lamaze International (natural childbirth):
800-368-4404

March of Dimes Birth Defects Foundation:
888-663-4637

National Herpes Hotline:
919-361-8488

National STD and AIDS Hotline:
800-227-8922

Sidelines National Support Network (high-risk pregnancy):
888-447-4754

Susan G. Komen Breast Cancer Foundation:
800-462-9273

CPSIA information can be obtained at www.ICGtesting.com
Printed in the USA
LVOW07s1630020715

444774LV00001B/22/P